Call the
Doctor

RONALD WHITE-COOPER was born in Grahamstown, South Africa, in 1892. He studied medicine at St Bartholomew's Hospital in London and served as a doctor on the Western Front between 1916 and 1918. He then worked at the South African Military Hospital in London, followed by a short period at Great Ormond Street Hospital for Sick Children, before becoming a GP in Dartmouth, Devon, in 1920. He practised as a doctor in Dartmouth and the surrounding area until 1949, when he returned to South Africa to work. He died in 1976. His memoirs were found in a trunk in the attic and edited by his granddaughter, Deborah White-Cooper, who is a trained journalist and worked as a television production executive.

Call the Doctor

A Country GP Between the Wars
Tales of Courage, Hardship and Hope

RONALD WHITE-COOPER

with DEBORAH WHITE-COOPER

PAN BOOKS

First published 2014 by Pan Books
an imprint of Pan Macmillan, a division of Macmillan Publishers Limited
Pan Macmillan, 20 New Wharf Road, London N1 9RR
Basingstoke and Oxford
Associated companies throughout the world
www.panmacmillan.com

ISBN 978-1-4472-5212-2

1 3 5 7 9 8 6 4 2

A CIP catalogue record for this book is available from the British Library.

Printed and bound by CPI Group (UK) Ltd, Croydon, CR0 4YY

Visit **www.panmacmillan.com** to read more about all our books
and to buy them. You will also find features, author interviews and
news of any author events, and you can sign up for e-newsletters
so that you're always first to hear about our new releases.

To Grandad, with love

Author's Note

In his memoirs, my grandfather mostly
referred to his patients as Mr X, Mrs Y and so on.
This would be rather confusing in a book and so
I have given his patients fictitious names.

Contents

Prologue
Grandad's Stories

Ninety-nine, ninety-nine, ninety-nine . . .

'Grandad . . . why do I have to say "ninety-nine" while you listen to my chest?'

It was one warm Sunday afternoon and I was sitting with my grandfather on his favourite lounger on the veranda of his home in Somerset West, South Africa. I had been suffering from a cold for a few days and my mother was worried that I was developing a wheezy cough.

'Ah, do you know, my dear, one of my patients once asked me the exact same question. Her name was Mrs Finch and she had a very bad case of bronchitis. Old Mrs Finch lived in England, in a very beautiful rural area just outside of Dartmouth, the town where I lived and practised for almost thirty years. She said that she'd much rather say "toasted cheese" or "pickled onions" – two of her favourite things to eat.'

I giggled and tried to push the cold metal plate of the stethoscope away from my skin. 'What did you say to her?'

'"Well," I said, "it's this way, Mrs Fitch. When I listen to your chest with my stethoscope – you know, this funny instrument – I listen to the resonance of the voice sounds coming from your lungs, and these sounds tell me whether or not your lung is healthy. Now, of all the words in the English language, 'ninety-nine' resonates best. Should you say unpleasant things, such as 'income tax', 'dustbins' or even the number 'ninety-eight', I would hear little that would help me in diagnosing your case. So 'ninety-nine' it has to be. This is just one of the tests we do to gain information about what is going on inside your chest." And then I gave old Mrs Finch a little bottle of medicine containing paregoric (camphorated tincture of opium), which smells strongly of liquorice and to which she was rather partial, and she wheezed out of my surgery satisfied and in the happiest of moods.'

'Oh,' I said, slightly daunted by the long words and the mention of medicine. 'What's going on inside *my* chest then?'

'A little high-pitched jingle caused by your cold but it's nothing serious. I think you'll be as right as rain in a few days.'

'So I won't need any medicine then?'

'No,' he smiled. 'But I shall prescribe a story to help the recovery process along a little.'

I curled myself into his side, taking care not to knock his bad leg.

'Once upon a time . . . '

I ALWAYS LOVED listening to my grandfather's stories. He was a natural storyteller and I put this down to his genuine and profound fascination with every person he encountered through his personal life and throughout his work as a doctor. As a child, he would entertain me with tales of interesting ailments, eccentric characters and the emergencies of ordinary people – of soldiers, grandmothers and babies.

After my grandfather's death, we discovered among his papers in a trunk in the attic a collection of stories he had written about his life as a doctor, starting in 1910 when he became a medical student to 1965 when he retired. Though rich in detail and dialogue, his notes were in no particular order and rather vaguely dated – presumably because he wrote them in later life, many years after the events they describe had taken place. So I looked for clues in the conditions and treatments he wrote about, as well as his descriptions of his patients' characters, their lives and their conversations, and created a timeline based on historical events and medical fact. Drawing on my own personal memories of him as well as those of other family members, I began to piece together the story of his extraordinary life. In it there are tales of shellfire, rats and slums in London a century ago; memories of the Great War when he tended the wounded at the front; and many varied accounts from his time as a GP in Devon, during the interwar years, the Second World War and beyond.

The recollections my grandfather left for us in his trunk are also a unique historical record of daily life in the medical profession during these harsh but innovative years. He witnessed huge medical advances during his lifetime. When he started practising there were no antibiotics, and the anaesthetic agents available were limited to chloroform, ether and a rather primitive array of drugs such as opium and morphine. How he must have wished Fleming's discovery of penicillin in 1928 had preceded the Great War, during which he embarked on his medical career – how many lives it could have saved. He saw the eradication of many diseases that he had previously treated on a daily basis, such as syphilis and tuberculosis, thanks to immunizations, new drugs and the introduction of public-health schemes tackling the lack of basic hygiene. Mental illness was also becoming better understood. Traumatic stress, or shell-shock as it was first classified, was originally linked to the more sophisticated artillery used in battle during the First World War; 80,000 British soldiers were diagnosed with shell-shock by the time the war ended, and approximately 346 were executed by firing squad for desertion or cowardice.

Much rarer mental conditions, such as Munchausen's syndrome by proxy, had not even been identified, let alone recognized – and my grandfather was perplexed when he first encountered such a case himself. However, increased knowledge and awareness, combined with the expanding use of technology and improved scientific techniques such as X-rays, gradually made diagnosis and treatment easier and more effective. To be a medical man in such times must have been very challenging, but so many discoveries and breakthroughs must also have made it incredibly exciting and rewarding.

It was not just the discovery of life-saving medicines that represented progress. Dispensing chemists as we know them today were rare, especially in rural areas. For much of my grandfather's early career as a GP he prepared all his own pre-scriptions and herbal medicines, though he did once claim to have known a pharmacist in Dartmouth called Mr Killer – so perhaps this was another reason! And getting about had been, in the early twentieth century, an achievement in itself. At the start of his career my grandfather visited his patients in a horse and trap, and yet by the end of his professional life, man was but a few years from walking on the moon and my grandfather was attending house calls in an automatic Chrysler motor car – one giant leap for mankind indeed.

His recollections are frequently poignant and moving. This was life in Britain during a time of huge sacrifice and hardship. It may have been an age of emotional reserve and the 'stiff upper lip', but in his accounts we see a doctor's extraordinary humanity and dedication to his patients – whether they were fellow soldiers on the front line or the enemy, or those in the wider community whom he served as a GP. As a doctor in a small rural town, it would have been almost impossible not to get to know your patients well, along with their families and personal circumstances, and it would therefore have been only natural for him to develop close friendships with those he treated. And alongside this deep-rooted sense of fellowship – the overwhelming belief that we're all in this together – lies a very British humour, making his stories for the most part an uplifting tribute to tough times.

His main practice during 1920–49 was in Dartmouth, and he also held surgeries in outlying villages and operated at the Dartmouth & Kingswear Hospital. In those days doctors were on call 24/7; no weekend passed uninterrupted, and my father recalls many a time when my grandfather would quietly let himself into the house before breakfast, tired and dishevelled after sitting through the night with an ailing patient. Perhaps it was his own tragic experience of bereavement that gave him such empathy with, and understanding of, his patients' needs.

Some twenty years after his time in Devon, when he and my grandmother had moved to South Africa, he wrote a letter to the *Dartmouth Chronicle* asking any of his old patients to get in touch. He received more than 300 letters from those he had looked after, as well as from some of those he had brought into the world during his thirty years as a Devonshire doctor. He apparently replied to each and every letter.

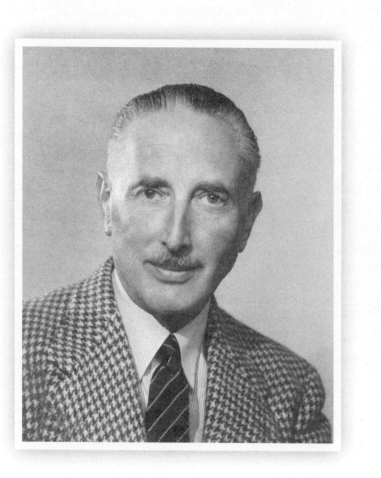

1

A Drop o' Gin 'to Keep
Me Spirits Up'

A Medical Student at Barts

IT WAS SEPTEMBER 1910 and I was on my way to the inaugural lecture at St Bartholomew's Hospital. Every new medical student was expected to attend, and that year our numbers exceeded all previous records. We filled the largest lecture theatre at Barts, tier upon tier, and expectantly awaited the arrival of the Dean of the hospital, who was to deliver his welcome speech. His entrance caused a sudden lull in the excited chatter – you could have heard a pin drop. He stood silently for a few minutes, looking up and scanning the numerous student faces peering intently down at him.

'Good God! What is going to become of all you gentlemen?' he began.

We were not exactly cheered by his address that day, as he spoke of the challenges that lay ahead, but his words of warning

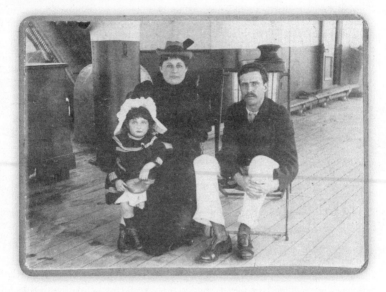

Aged three years old, with my mother and father, January 1896.

were not enough to dim my enthusiasm. You see, I had always wanted to be a doctor.

Once, when I was a boy, I found a dead chameleon in our garden. I carefully placed the little corpse in a tin box and buried it. About a year later I dug the tin up, and inside was a perfect little skeleton, which I duly dismantled. At the time my family and I were living in Grahamstown in South Africa, which is where I was born on 23 August 1892. Although my father, William White-Cooper, was English, he had emigrated to the Cape in 1890 for health reasons, as he suffered from a hearing disorder and it was hoped the drier air would benefit him. A year later he met and married my mother, Amy Hess, who with her parents had also emigrated to the Cape from Frankfurt in Germany. I had two younger brothers – Rupert who was born in 1895, followed by Denis in 1899. Sadly, my sister Evelyn died in 1894, when she was less than a year old.

In those days Grahamstown, which is located in the Eastern Cape, was a small but thriving city with a predominantly British population – this influence was evident in all its colonial-style buildings and residences. Also known as the 'City of Saints', on account of the number of churches, it was the perfect place for my father to set up practice as an architect. He became particularly well known for his designs, in red brick, of prominent schools and public buildings, such as St Andrew's College, Kingswood School and the Training College.

We lived a happy, peaceful existence, and though the second Boer War of 1899–1902 raged all around us, it seemed a world apart from the one we knew. However, we couldn't

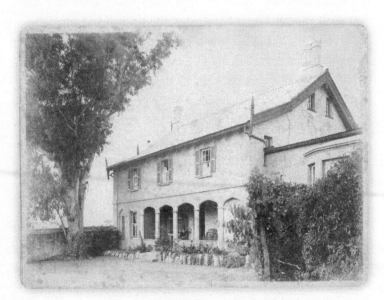

'The Retreat': my family home in Grahamstown, 1902.

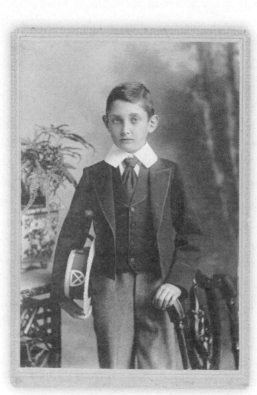

Aged nine years old, November 1901.

escape it entirely. I recall one Easter Sunday when our family was attending the morning service at St George's Cathedral, the city's largest Anglican church, where I was a choir boy. Suddenly during prayers the Drostdy Arch bell began to ring loudly and numerous hooters sounded. Immediately we rushed out of our pews, spilling out of the church and onto the street. British Army scouts outside informed us that a Boer commando – some 500 strong – had been sighted fifteen miles from the town. There was much excitement and the British town guard, of which my father was a member, was immediately called up to man the trenches, which had already been dug around Grahamstown as a precaution. I remember him putting on his cartridge belt – known as a bandolier – and then marching purposefully off, a Martini-Henry rifle resting on his shoulder. Fortunately the Boers left us alone, and subsequently we heard that their commandant was General Jan Smuts, who later became Prime Minister of South Africa.

I also remember there being a Boer prisoner-of-war camp at the end of our street – Prince Alfred Street – and I would often see a string of very dishevelled prisoners shuffling along, escorted by mounted British troops.

IN SEPTEMBER 1906, aged fourteen, I was sent on the HMS *Kildonan Castle* to England, where I was to take up a place as a boarder at Marlborough College school in Wiltshire. During exeats (the holidays) I stayed with my Uncle George in Courtfield Gardens, opposite Gloucester Road Underground station, in London. He was a highly respected physician at St George's

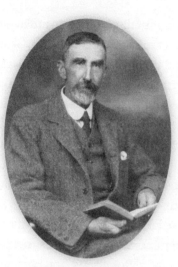

Uncle George.

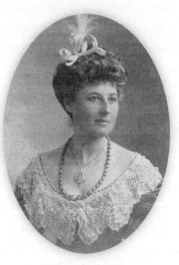

My mother, 1908.

Hospital and I greatly enjoyed listening to his stories of life in a large London teaching hospital.

My three and a half years at Marlborough were not particularly happy for me. I had never lived away from home before, let alone in a land so distant, and I missed my family and old school friends dreadfully. I found life in an English boarding school very different from what I was used to, and I took some time to settle in. I did, however, become very friendly with a boy called Alex Sim, whose father was the vicar of Lower Brixham in Devon, and I was always made to feel very welcome at their family home. We spent many happy school holidays together and, during these visits, I grew particularly fond of Alex's cousin, Rosamund Tracey, who was about five years younger than us. She lived with her parents and younger brother in nearby Dartmouth, where her father was vicar of St Saviour's Church. Rosamund was great fun, with a terrific sense of humour and an infectious giggle, and I was always delighted when she joined us for games of croquet and tennis, or for a picnic on the beach.

In 1910, during the Easter holidays, I returned to South Africa for a short visit. What made my stay particularly unforgettable was the appearance of Halley's Comet – after an absence of seventy-five years. I watched it flash brightly from my bedroom window and made a small sketch of it, which my mother proudly hung in the parlour.

Back at school, I studied hard for exams, gaining the results I needed to go to medical college, and in September 1910, aged eighteen, I enrolled as a student at St Bartholomew's Hospital in the City of London. My grandfather, also called William White-Cooper, who was Queen Victoria's oculist, had studied there, and I felt proud to be following in his footsteps and in those of many other eminent medical men. On my first day I stood, awestruck, in front of the grand arched stone entrance to the oldest hospital in England. Then I wandered through the hospital's impressive buildings, some dating back to the reign of Henry VIII, marvelling at the artworks hanging on the walls of the grand staircase, illustrating the biblical stories of the Good Samaritan and the 'Healing of the Sick at the Pool of Bethesda', which had been painted especially for the hospital by the famous artist William Hogarth.

In those days London medical students were a happy and carefree lot, and life in one of the big teaching hospitals was always interesting and varied. We were expected to complete five years' study for a professional qualification, and this meant attending all lectures, classes and demonstrations on different branches of medicine, where our presence – or absence – was duly noted by a zealous hospital porter.

Accommodation was provided and we slept and ate all our meals in residential quarters in nearby Little Britain, a street that formed the northern boundary of the hospital.

One met all types at Barts. There were those who were serious about their studies and others who were just out for a good time; and there were even those who considered getting into the Hospital 1st XV rugby team far more important than scholastic achievements. Most were between the ages of twenty and twenty-five, but a few were middle-aged. There was a retired Indian army colonel and a retired bank manager, a Jamaican (who was an excellent musician), an Egyptian and a Senegalese.

There was also a South African, who I suppose could be called the star student, as he had already been at the hospital for seven years. He apparently had no wish to qualify as he found student life far too pleasant and rewarding and, as his family was well off, he had no desperate need to practise medicine for a living. Despite this, he regularly took the examination papers and, when it came to the oral examinations, he was the bane of the examiners and thoroughly enjoyed pulling their legs. During one test the examiner held up a skull and pointed to the opening in its base, through which the spinal cord would pass.

'Please explain what goes through this hole,' he said.

'I know many a good pint passes through there, sir!' came the student's cheeky reply.

That was the last time he was permitted to attend an oral examination, though he was still a student when I left the hospital some five years later.

AT ST BARTHOLOMEW'S HOSPITAL one of the highlights of the medical student's calendar was View Day – an annual open day, which dates back to the founding of the hospital in 1123. Historically it was an inspection of the hospital by the Treasurer and governors, but in time it also became an opportunity for family, friends and other visitors to look round the hospital. The Pathological Museum and Pharmaceutical Department were by far the most popular sites, especially as they were not generally open to members of the public. In the latter one could see the manufacture of tablets and various medicines; there were also leeches swimming around in glass bowls. In those days leeches were still used to relieve congestion.

Most, if not all, London hospitals possess a museum, which as a rule displays pathological specimens pickled in jars containing spirit or formalin. Barts was no exception. There were rare specimens of inflamed tissues and growths, and there were freaks and monsters in large bottles who, had they lived, might have graced a Barnum & Bailey circus show and made a lot of money for the owner. I particularly remember one: a baby that was a true Cyclops, born with an eye in the centre of its forehead and with a nose and mouth resembling a pig snout – it really was an extraordinary case. In my practice I occasionally delivered children with various anatomical deformities: cleft palate, hare-lip, clubbed feet, spina bifida and imperforate anus; but I have never seen or heard of a Cyclops since. In another jar was the head of a lunatic who had apparently cut off his own nose with a straight razor. The story went that a handy warden rushed up to the man, seized the razor from him, picked up the amputated nose and quickly pressed it back into position, where it was later strapped with plaster. The portion that had been cut off grew back again, but it was not quite straight and you could see the scar of the line of separation quite clearly in the specimen.

Also on display was a motley array of surgical instruments with wooden, bone and ivory handles – crude tools of every description. When one considers the stainless-steel instruments in use today, it makes one shudder to think of the wretched patients undergoing operations in medieval times without even an anaesthetic. There were also fearsome-looking amputation saws. The victims of an amputation operation, we were told, were completely drunk on rum and were held down on the table by half a dozen hospital porters. Next, the offending limb would be amputated, and then the stump immersed in boiling pitch to seal the wound.

Another curious relic was a leather apron that appeared to be covered in layer upon layer of dried blood. It must have been worn to protect the surgeon's clothing – not for the benefit of the unfortunate patient. Instead of being washed and cleaned after use, it must have been thrown onto a peg dripping with blood, until such time as it was needed again. How the patients ever survived these operations remains a complete mystery. Sepsis and septicaemia must have been rampant, as antibacterials and antiseptics were unknown in those days.

HAVING PASSED FIRST-YEAR examinations in the subjects of Chemistry, Physics and Biology, the student next embarked on Anatomy and Physiology. To most students unaccustomed to seeing a corpse, it was quite a shock when one first entered the Anatomy Department, for laid out on steel tables were some dozen dead bodies, both male and female. I gathered that these were generally unclaimed bodies from local workhouses, but on occasion people left their bodies to the hospital for the benefit of medical progress.

As a rule, four to six students were allocated to each body – one dissecting an upper limb, one a lower limb, another the head and neck, another the thorax and abdomen. Prior to being dissected, the arteries of each body were injected with a solution of red lead, so that they could easily be seen during the dissection. Anatomy fascinated me. I carried out some intricate dissections and at the end of the year became a pro-sector – the person with the special task of preparing a dis-section for demonstration – and was awarded the Treasurer's Prize in Junior Practical Anatomy. Had I known precisely what this entailed, I would certainly not have wished to win this prize, because it meant that I was required to prepare all the dissections for the hospital museum (which were later bottled in jars of spirit), and as these dissections were mostly carried out on Saturday afternoons I missed many a good game of hockey in the winter and of tennis in the summer.

After the day's work the various arms, legs and other body parts were carried out to a room at the back of the hospital and placed in large tanks of formalin to preserve them. I am afraid that by the end of the term, the various tanks contained a thorough mix-up of anatomical parts: Mr X's legs, Mrs V's arms and Mrs D's chest and abdomen. In the years to come, special laws would be introduced to govern this area of medicine and medical colleges would enforce much stricter rules, whereby dissected body parts would be labelled to avoid confusion and to enable proper burials, but this was not the case when I was studying anatomy, and I never discovered where the remains of these unfortunate people were sent at the end of the year.

The well-known expression 'boys will be boys' was never more apt than amongst us medical students. While we took our studies seriously, we also greatly enjoyed a good prank, and on one occasion my friends and I attached a length of catgut to the penis of a cadaver awaiting dissection. We threaded it through an eyelet in the ceiling and took the end of the line with us into a nearby cupboard, where we waited impatiently. For an hour or so much merriment ensued whenever any unsuspecting person entered the Dissection Room and we would give the cord a vigorous yank!

IN MY THIRD YEAR I attended lectures on pharmacology, during which our professor used to give us practical demonstrations on the effects of various drugs – one week atropine, another week morphine, another cocaine, and so on. As a rule cats, dogs, guinea pigs or mice were used in these demonstrations. The doses were usually not enough to kill the unfortunate creatures, but were strong enough to demonstrate the effects of the drug. This particular week our professor said, 'Today gentlemen, one of *you* is going to be my guinea pig, for I am going to demonstrate the signs and symptoms of nicotine-poisoning, which in large doses can produce death. Now, I want a non-smoker to volunteer.'

At the time, as it happened, I was a non-smoker – the only one in the class, and a fact of which I was rather proud. However, I quickly regretted it. All eyes were on me as I stood up and made my way to the front of the room.

'Come along,' said the professor, 'sit down on this chair and make yourself comfortable. I should like you to remove your coat and shirt, so that we can examine your heart and lungs and fix a blood-pressure manometer to your arm.'

Having done this, and much to the amusement of my fellow students, I was given the rankest cigar imaginable, which the professor kindly lit for me. 'Draw away,' he said, 'and take some really deep breaths.'

A needle on a revolving drum – an early version of the electrocardiogram machine that is in use nowadays – traced my heartbeats, and my blood pressure was being tested at frequent intervals.

'Now,' said the professor, 'you will notice the sudden pallor on our friend's face. He is beginning to perspire – can't you see the beads of perspiration on his forehead? I will take his blood pressure. It is coming down, in delightful fashion. How are you feeling, old chap,' he asked me, 'not too good eh?'

'I am beginning to feel a little nauseous.'

'Don't worry about that – we have a large basin ready for you under your chair. Now, gentlemen, you will notice that his pulse is quickening, and his heartbeats are slightly irregular. His blood pressure is dropping beautifully, and he is salivating – always a precursor to vomiting. How are you feeling now?'

'I feel sick and dizzy – yes, I want to be sick,' I gulped.

'Wouldn't you like to take a few more puffs before you are?'

'No, definitely not – I want to be sick right now,' I said, reaching desperately for the basin.

'Oh well,' said the professor happily. 'Gentlemen, you have seen a perfect demonstration of the ill-effects of nicotine-poisoning – our subject has produced them all: pallor, sweating, salivation, drop in blood pressure, irregular heartbeat, quickened pulse, nausea and vomiting. Thank you for your excellent cooperation,' he said, patting me on the back.

IN 1913, ON MY TWENTY-FIRST BIRTHDAY, I made a trip back to South Africa to celebrate with family and friends. My parents had recently moved to Cradock, a small farming town in the Karoo area of the Eastern Cape, where my father continued to run a successful architectural practice.

One afternoon, my brother Denis was taken ill and the family doctor, Dr Karl Bremer, who later became the Minister of Health in South Africa, was called to the house. My mother duly introduced me as a young medical student, and when Dr Bremer asked whether I would like to join him on his rounds and observe operations at the local hospital, I agreed with great enthusiasm. A few days later he visited again and said to me, 'Here, young fellow, I want *you* to administer an anaesthetic at an emergency operation.'

'But, Dr Bremer, I know nothing about anaesthetics. I have only just completed my third year and haven't yet attended demonstrations on anaesthesia,' I told him.

'Don't panic,' he replied, 'I will give you a bottle of chloroform and a mask and tell you exactly what to do.'

He explained that this was a most unusual case, as the patient was a young native woman living in a kraal – a traditional African village of thatched huts – some seven miles out

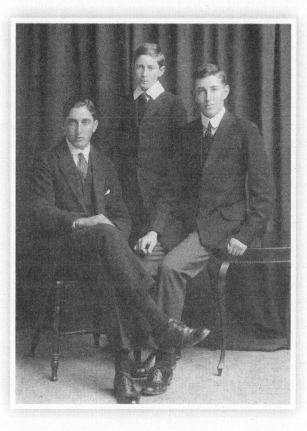

With my brothers, Rupert and Denis (right) *in Cradock, 1913.*

of Cradock. 'She is much too ill to move, so we shall have to go and operate on her in her hut this evening,' he told me.

First we travelled to the hospital to fetch some sterile sheets and sterile operating instruments, along with four candles and some bottles to stick them in. We also took a bottle of chloroform and a mask.

That evening we set off at about six o'clock and, having opened and closed a dozen farm gates on the way, we finally reached the village, by which time it was dark. We lit the candles and spread a sterile sheet on the floor of the hut, which was made of dried cattle-dung polished smooth. We lifted the patient carefully and Dr Bremer put on a sterile gown, while I was given the chloroform and mask.

'Now,' said Dr Bremer, 'if you want to kill the patient, place thirty drops of chloroform onto the mask and clamp down on the patient's face. If, on the other hand, you do not wish to commit murder, you proceed like this. Drop two drops on the mask and count five seconds. Then drop three drops and count five seconds, and so on. By the time the patient is inhaling ten drops, I shall begin operating.'

A gangrenous appendix was duly removed and the patient made a full recovery.

During the same holiday I began to nurture an interest in collecting beetles – *Coleoptera*, as the genus is known. I spent many an hour wandering out in the open grasslands of the veldt, watching dung beetles hard at work. It was fascinating to see the male beetle rolling a ball of dung along; and then the female, who should be helping, would sometimes crawl onto the ball and take a rest, which naturally impeded its progress. The female lays her egg in the centre of the ball, and here it remains buried until heat hatches it. The little grub then feeds its way from the centre of the ball to the outside world.

When it was time for me to return to London to continue my medical training, I mounted some of these beetles on a piece of card and brought them back with me, whereupon I presented them to the Natural History Museum in South Kensington. To my utter astonishment, I was told I had discovered several new species.

THE INTER-HOSPITAL rugby matches were the highlight of the winter season, and pitched battles would be fought by opposing students on the field, before the commencement of every game. Many hospitals had a special mascot. Guy's Hospital had a large milk churn painted with the hospital's colours, which was suspended from the cross-bar of the goal post. St Thomas's mascot was a cannon, while King's College had a lion. Another hospital, I seem to recall, had a wooden figurehead resembling Cleopatra, which at one time must have graced the bow of an old-time sailing ship.

It was during an inter-hospital hockey match, in early 1914, that I sustained a painful injury, which developed into synovitis, an inflammation of the synovial membrane enveloping the knee – commonly known as 'water on the knee' – and which led to me being admitted to Barts as a patient. Having previously walked the wards with some dignity, I was now helplessly wheeled into the hospital's Henry Ward, but it was interesting to see the workings of a large London hospital from a patient's point of view (previously I had only known them as a dresser or clerk, both of which were supervised junior house roles and part of our medical curriculum).

There were about twenty-six beds in this ward, and the sister in charge – who wore a blue uniform and white cap – was a strict disciplinarian who stood no nonsense. In fact she might be called a real dragon, for students as well as nurses went in fear of her. The day began at the unearthly hour of 5 a.m., with the night and day staff seeing to one's ablutions and to the making of beds. The ward sister would read morning prayers. Breakfast followed – and ample it was, too. Next came along the ward cleaners and floor polishers. A paper boy would deliver the daily paper and a barber would stop by and enquire whether you wished to be shaved or would shave yourself. By the time we had finished reading the daily news, the medical students would come along – each to his assigned patients – and your case history would be reviewed and written down on notes, which were hung at the end of your bed. A little later lunch was served and afterwards, at about 1.30 p.m., the great surgeon and his team of dressers would stream into the ward accompanied by the ward sister and a blue-belt nurse, who wore a blue-and-white-striped uniform. Each bed would be visited, one by one, and when it was my turn, I would get my fair share of leg-pulling. Lights went out early, after evening prayers, which were once again led by the ward sister.

Being a light sleeper, I did not enjoy the nights. I was continually woken by the grunts, snores or coughs of my fellow patients. However, this was compensated for during the day by the pleasure I took from talking to my fellow bedmates. On my left was a butcher from nearby Smithfield Meat Market, and on my right a rather lugubrious fellow, who I found out was an undertaker (though he preferred to be called a 'funeral director'). I fully sympathized with him, but imagine that his eyes must have feasted on those poor mortals who were screened off in the ward, when about to depart from the world!

The butcher, who was a cheerful cockney and a champion snorer, told me illuminating tales of the hundreds of sewer rats that abounded in the meat market, when the men came to work in the early hours of the morning; and of how these rats nibbled at the meat lying about and then scuttled away and disappeared down the drains as soon as the workers arrived.

Visiting days were, of course, the highlight of the week. The flower seller outside the Henry VIII gate, at the hospital entrance, would do a roaring trade as mothers and fathers, husbands and wives bought bouquets of flowers, as well as magazines and periodicals. And for two hours just twice a week – on Wednesdays and Sundays – the wards in the hospital would buzz with laughter and animated conversation.

ONCE BACK ON MY FEET, I continued with my studies, attending classes and lectures on surgery, vaccination and public health, as well as demonstrations on anaesthesia and medical and surgical morbid anatomy and pathology – all subjects that I greatly enjoyed. I also spent a month or so as a dresser in both the gynaecological and ophthalmic wards, where I assisted surgeons on their rounds by writing up case notes and by dressing minor surgical cases under supervision. For a few weeks during my final summer session I spent some time at a lunatic asylum, where I observed unfortunate cases of insanity – another subject that I found particularly fascinating.

During my career as a doctor I must have delivered well over 3,000 babies. As a medical student I was very pleased to attend lectures and demonstrations in midwifery and gynaecology, held in the hospital's Elizabeth Maternity Ward. There was plenty of practical training as well, and each student was expected to do three weeks on the 'district'. This involved attending an average twenty confinements.

Our hospital's 'district' in those days was the sordid slum area around Smithfield Meat Market, one of London's oldest markets. My work took me along narrow cobbled streets with evil-smelling drains, through dingy passages and up rickety stairs, into gloomy rooms lit by a single candle. The rooms were often ill ventilated – the foul smell of poverty all-pervading and never to be forgotten.

On many occasions the room to which I was called was almost bare: no rugs or carpets, the window framed by a pathetic dirty curtain. The only pieces of furniture were often a double bed, a small table and a chair. The hospital would provide sheets, blankets, hot-water bottles, cotton wool, sanitary towels and other necessities for the more impoverished cases. Some of the poorer families lived in one large room, such was the overcrowding in these double-storeyed tenements, and I frequently had to send children into the streets while their mother was adding to the family. One of the things that struck me was how a wizened, miserable-looking mother often produced a fine, strapping infant of nine or ten pounds, although within a few weeks that same babe would lose many ounces in weight, owing to the poor quality of its mother's milk or to errors in feeding. Anyway, nature at least appeared to give all the babies a good start in life.

Some of the midwives I encountered were Dickensian characters, sitting with folded arms at the end of the bed dispensing 'motherly' advice to the wretched mother-to-be during labour pain.

''Ere, dearie, yer pulls on that rope, see – each time that pain comes on,' they'd say, having tied a stout rope at the end of the bed. If the poor mother shouted out in pain, the midwife would often add, 'Now come along, dearie, yer've 'ad yer pleasure, see – now yer going to 'ave yer pain.'

And how those midwives loved a drop of gin, often sending one of the children on errands to the pub around the corner for sixpenny-worth of the spirit. 'Just to keep me spirits up!' they would protest loudly. And how they loved to gossip: Mrs Malcolm had had two sets of twins in just over a year; Mrs Reid had had five miscarriages, but was still hoping; and Mrs Smith's husband was a real 'bad 'un', always on the drink, and the children near-starving.

Their rooms were often running with vermin, and I felt compelled to have an antiseptic bath on my return to hospital quarters. It was amazing how few cases of childbirth fever we saw, considering the primitive conditions under which we had to work. Lysol disinfectant and carbolic soap were our two mainstays, and of course we wore rubber gloves and sterile gowns. Instruments and forceps, when required, were boiled by spirit lamp in the copper sterilizer that I always carried with me.

I can remember my fear and trepidation the first time I applied forceps. Having anaesthetized the mother with a drop of chloroform, I had to pretend to her and to the midwife that I was an expert. Having only practised the art on a hospital dummy, I must have appeared proficient at least and felt much relieved, or my reputation would have sunk to zero.

When we were in real trouble, with a post-partum haemorrhage or obstructed labour, we would quickly send the husband or a neighbour on a bicycle to the hospital with a towel, on which a cross was daubed in the patient's blood. This was for the resident obstetric superintendent and was code for 'Come immediately: I am in dire trouble'!

I thoroughly enjoyed my time in the 'district' and greatly admired the courage of many of the poorly nourished women – and their marvellous cockney humour, in spite of the hard lives they led. I doubt if they ever visited the cinema or the theatre; their life revolved around the pub or street-corner gossip. They were a class that seems to have vanished today since the great improvement in modern living standards.

At the end of my studies I was very pleased to win the hospital's Matthews Duncan Prize for Midwifery and Gynaecology. I seriously considered specializing in these subjects, but the First World War intervened.

THE SUMMER OF 1914 was a particularly fine one. I spent my holidays with friends in Sussex and, apart from being blown up in a steam car and deposited in a hedgerow when the engine boiler overheated, the world seemed happy and at peace. These were halcyon days; income tax was negligible, the British Empire ruled the world and Britannia ruled the seas. Then, all of a sudden, the papers splashed news of the assassination of the Austrian Crown Prince at Sarajevo by a Serbian nationalist on 28 June. War clouds quickly gathered, as Austria invaded Serbia in July, and her ally Germany invaded Belgium and Luxembourg and headed towards France. Britain, who was allied with France, was forced to take action. At midnight on 4 August, Britain was at war with Germany. Within a matter of weeks, it seemed, the world as we knew it was turned upside down.

I well remember the excitement of that night. A number of my medical student friends and I took a bus to Whitehall, where the streets were teeming with straw-hatted crowds and Union Jacks were everywhere to be seen. Regular uniformed soldiers, when found, were triumphantly paraded shoulder-high through the streets, and the air was filled with cries of 'God Save the King' and other patriotic songs. We gradually wended our way to Piccadilly Circus and eventually ended up at the Cafe Royal. There pandemonium ruled, as all the German waiters had been severely mauled and had therefore fled. It was a madhouse and, as there was no one left to serve us, we wandered back onto the streets and soon lost ourselves in the seething mass of humanity.

Young men, eager to fight for King and country, were soon joining the army in large numbers, but we medical students were told to continue with our studies. Then, in early 1915, the Admiralty made an application for senior medical students to join the navy as surgical probationers, whereupon four of my friends and I decided to apply. Although we had not yet completed our medical curriculum, we were medically examined, found fit and ordered to go to Gieves, the military tailors, to collect our uniforms.

For several days we proudly paraded the streets and attended hospital in our naval uniforms, with the little squiggle of gold and red braid adorning our sleeves. Then one morning we each found a long blue envelope bearing our name on the breakfast table. It was postmarked 'Admiralty', with an anchor printed in the corner of the envelope. Thinking these were our orders for posting to a ship, we hurriedly ripped open our letters. But our spirits quickly sank, for the letter advised us that the policy had changed and, due to a shortage of naval surgeons, we were to return our uniforms to Messrs Gieves without delay and go back to hospital to get qualified – as soon as possible.

2

'There's a Ghost in the Mortuary!'

A House Physician at Barts

MY LAST YEAR as a medical student seemed to pass quickly and, on successfully completing my final examinations during the summer of 1915, the next six months at St Bartholomew's Hospital were some of the happiest in my life. I was fortunate in gaining a six-month appointment as house physician under Dr Morley Fletcher – a most-revered general physician at the hospital. Considering the fierce competition for these places, this was quite an achievement. In all there were a dozen of us housemen at Barts and each day we gathered around the fountain in the Hospital Square awaiting the arrival of our 'chief', whom, along with our dressers and medical clerks, we accompanied on his ward rounds. We had a rota for being on duty in the casualty wards, where all through the day and often at night we attended urgent accident or medical cases, which – when necessary – would be admitted to the hospital.

It was shortly afterwards that I received my first medical fee: for giving evidence in a suicide case. Every doctor, in the course of a long medical career, comes across suicides or attempted suicides, in one form or another. These may be due to a cut throat, a shooting, coal-gas poisoning, an overdose of sleeping tablets, motor-car exhaust fumes or poisoning. I have, unfortunately, had experience of them all. This particular case was one of self-inflicted phosphorus-poisoning and it had a peculiar sequel. The patient, a middle-aged woman, made herself sandwiches onto which she spread – instead of jam – a thick layer of rat poison. She was unconscious upon admission and smelt strongly of wax vestas (or matches as they are called nowadays). Within twenty-four hours she had become jaundiced and her urine was luminous in the dark. In spite of all our efforts, she died.

In due course she was placed in the mortuary, along with other dead bodies. Now it so happened that every evening a hospital orderly by the name of Harry went up to the mortuary to open the ventilating shafts. One evening several of us house-men were sitting in the Hospital Square after dinner when Harry rushed up to us, his face quite pale and his eyes bulging.

'I have seen one, I have seen one!' he yelled. 'There's a ghost in the mortuary – it's awful!'

Well, we all jumped up and hurried along to investigate and, as we opened the mortuary door, we saw that my phosphorus-patient's body was completely luminous in the dark, and a shimmering green light appeared to be rising from her body. There was no need to turn on the electric light, for her body lit up all the other corpses lying on adjoining slabs. It was certainly an eerie sight, and it was no wonder that poor Harry had such a fright.

Coincidentally I had another case of phosphorus-poisoning just a few months later, and although this patient became slightly jaundiced, owing to the harmful effect of this poison on the liver, she made a full recovery. But of course the problem with treating an attempted suicide is that successful treatment does not always meet with the patient's approval. In one case of mine a middle-aged lady, slightly unhinged, who lived an unhappy life with her sister and brother-in-law, took an overdose of sleeping tablets and was admitted to hospital in an unconscious state to have her stomach washed out. It so happened that in the morning I was on my hospital rounds when she woke. Seeing me at the end of her bed, she groaned, 'Oh no, it's you, is it . . . ? I had hoped to see St Peter!'

LIFE AS A HOUSEMAN was interesting and varied and there was great fellowship between us. We were a cheery bunch, and our Jamaican friend would entertain us with his musical talent – he was a wizard on the piano!

About a month before Christmas the housemen and their clerks began looking for talent for the Christmas concert. Groups were formed, as concert parties for the entertainment of the patients, and there was a friendly rivalry between these parties as they frolicked from ward to ward. In fact Christmas time in a London hospital is a time of jovial festivities and happiness. It is strange how the numbers of outpatients swell significantly a few days before Christmas, with real or feigned illnesses – the prospective patients hoping to be admitted in time to receive a present from the huge Christmas tree erected in each ward and partake of the Yuletide lunch of turkey and plum pudding.

Although we housemen were a gay and friendly bunch, we had one unpopular member. This individual had the unpleasant habit of barging into private get-togethers given by one or other of the housemen. In the beginning his uninvited intrusions were tolerated, but after a time he became a real nuisance. It was well known that he revelled in chocolate eclairs, which he ate with real gusto. Word went round the breakfast table in our college dining room one morning that so-and-so was giving a special tea party that afternoon. Feeling certain that our uninvited friend would duly make an appearance, a number of chocolate eclairs were suitably doctored with heavy doses of calomel powder – a violent laxative. Sure enough, at about 4.30 p.m., there was a knock at the door and in came the uninvited guest, making suitable apologies and excuses, but nevertheless intending to stay and partake of the delicious eats. In due course two eclairs disappeared and, shortly before leaving, a third followed.

It was a very bleary-eyed, haggard-looking houseman who appeared at the breakfast table the next morning, complaining of a most frightful night, half of which had been spent in the lavatory. Had any of us a similar fate?

'No,' we replied, 'we are all in excellent health and slept quite peacefully.'

'Well, I must have caught a chill or have been poisoned,' he reasoned.

A few weeks later our friend, not having taken the hint, once again barged into a tea party. I wasn't present, but I was told this was just too much for the housemen concerned. That night this uninvited gentleman was frog-marched to the Hospital Square, where he was ceremoniously dumped in the fountain. He must at last have awakened to his ungentlemanly habits, because from that day on all intrusions to private parties ceased abruptly.

On our free Saturday evenings my fellow housemen and I would take a double-decker bus up to London's lively West End, to see a show. A popular meeting place in those days was the Leicester Lounge, or we would meet for supper in one of those little Soho restaurants – a favourite was Pinoli's – where for the modest sum of 2s. 6d. one could get a four-course dinner. I remember one menu distinctly: whitebait followed by devilled chicken legs. These legs were collected from the big hotels, like the Carlton and the Ritz, for their wealthy clientele fed only on the breast of chicken – no drumsticks for them! For a sweet we had Neapolitan ice cream, followed by cheese straws. It makes one's mouth water, when you compare present-day prices for a four-course dinner, but then of course this was in the years before the war.

After the meal we would patronize one of the West End shows. The most popular establishments at this time were the

London Pavilion, the Alhambra and the Hippodrome, where the comedians George Robey, Alfred Lester and Marie Lloyd and the stage beauties Lily Elsie, Phyllis Dare and Gertie Millar entertained and entranced audiences.

I was walking through Leicester Square one afternoon when I noticed a magician's shop – all sorts of tricks were displayed in the window. Having always been interested in conjuring, I entered the shop and there behind the counter was a little man, who looked so ill and pale that I said to him, 'You don't look at all well – are you sure you shouldn't see a doctor, or at least be resting in bed?'

'Not on your life,' he replied. 'No more hospital for me, I was discharged only yesterday. You would be surprised what those doctors did to me. My bowels are now like Clapham Junction – joined to my stomach in some miraculous manner. Anyway, thank goodness I have survived their experiments!'

'Well,' I said, 'I expect they did a short-circuiting of your stomach – what we call a gastric enterostomy or a partial gastrectomy. You see, I happen to be a doctor myself.'

'Well, I apologize,' he replied, 'if I have said anything derogatory against your fraternity, but I have been through hell. Now my greatest wish is to see this operation performed on someone else – would that be at all possible?'

'Yes, I don't see why not,' I said. 'Why don't you give me your telephone number and I will let you know when I see a similar case to yours on the daily operating list.'

In a few days one such case materialized, so I telephoned the little man and told him to be in the Hospital Square at

1.30 p.m. sharp. He turned up in good time, but looked so ill and forlorn that I hesitated, saying, 'Look, I really don't want to have to carry you out, should you faint. Are you sure you will be all right?'

'I don't mind a drop of blood,' he reassured me, and so we mounted the steps of the theatre and both peered down to watch the operation. 'Gee!' he said. 'Did they do all that to me?'

'Yes, I presume so,' I replied.

'Well, I never!' he said.

'Now, have you seen enough?' I asked, once the procedure was complete.

'Oh, is this the only operation, or am I able to see another?' the little man asked.

'No,' I said, 'they continue until 6 p.m., but I do not think you will care to see the next – an unfortunate woman is having a breast amputated for cancer.'

'I don't mind a drop of blood,' insisted the little man.

Not only did he sit through this operation, but two more after that. He appeared utterly riveted, but eventually, when it was 5 p.m., I suggested that he should come down to the students' restaurant and have a cup of tea with me. While we chatted he put his hand into his coat pocket, pulled out his wallet and handed me his visiting card – he was none other than Will Goldston, one of the greatest magicians of the day and a leading light at London's best-known Magicians' Club, which he had founded a few years earlier. Unknowingly I had been entertaining the High Priest of Magic.

'Now,' he went on, 'one good turn deserves another. You

have given me one of the most interesting afternoons I can recall. Here are two tickets. You see, we magicians meet once a month to show each other our new tricks and illusions. The whole audience naturally is made up of magicians, but you and a friend will be my special guests.'

So a week later I took my brother Rupert, who was then a student at the Bartlett School of Architecture at University College London, to watch a very exclusive show, and I am sure we enjoyed it far more than our little friend watching the art of surgery.

ALTHOUGH WE READ ABOUT the hostilities, such as the U-boat attacks on our shipping vessels and the Battle of Ypres, where chlorine gas was first used by the Germans with terrible effect, the world at war seemed far removed from the day-to-day reality of a busy London hospital. Until, that is, a cool September evening in 1915 – one I will never forget. It was a starlit night, with no moon visible, and we had just had supper in the hospital restaurant. I was one of the house doctors on duty that evening and, after dinner, several of us walked into the Hospital Square and sat down on a bench by the fountain, chatting animatedly and discussing the day's work. After a few minutes we heard the most curious whirring noise and then a distant explosion, accompanied by a flash of light in the sky. Not knowing what it was, we all ran up the stairs to the top of the pathology block, where we would get a better view.

We had barely reached the roof when we heard another strange swishing sound – then we were temporarily blinded by a brilliant white light and blown clean off our feet. Had it not been for a parapet around the roof, we would probably have been blown off the top of the building. This explosion was quickly followed by the crashing sound of hundreds of panes of glass falling in the square. The noise was indescribable and for a moment there was much confusion, as we did not know the source of the explosion. But within a short time searchlights picked out a huge silver, cigar-shaped object floating across the sky. Only then did we realize that it was a Zeppelin raid!

Visibly shaken, we all got up and shouted, 'Bomb!' Then we rushed down into the square, where shattered glass covered the ground. As we ventured towards the hospital gateway to Little Britain, near our residential quarters, we could see that a bomb had fallen in Bartholomew Close and there was a huge crater in front of a public house known to students as the 'Nipple'. Water mains were flooding the street.

Within a few minutes there were yet more booming sounds, which seemed to come from the other side of Smithfield Meat Market, and later on we heard that a bomb had fallen outside Liverpool Street Station, striking a motor bus and causing a number of fatalities. Shortly afterwards ambulances were bringing in the casualties – some critically injured, some with bomb fragments embedded in their bodies, others badly burned or struck with pieces of paving stone. We were operating on the wounded, young and old, until the early hours of the next morning.

The landlord of the 'Nipple' had evidently been standing outside, at the front of his pub, when the bomb fell. He was never seen again, but his leg – reputedly with his name on a sock – was recovered some days later, hanging up in one of the trees in the Hospital Square.

Meanwhile in the south wing of the hospital – in the Elizabeth Maternity Ward – the sudden shock started up all the expectant mothers with labour pains. One can imagine the pandemonium, especially with the cool night air blowing through the shattered maternity-ward windows – now without a pane of glass and no light.

The anti-aircraft gunfire was useless, for after all our gunners had little or no experience or previous practice, and any aerial gun shrapnel failed to get anywhere near the Zeppelin. The majestic-looking silver cigar continued to drift leisurely over London, dropping its lethal load at will and leaving death and destruction in its wake. Soon fires were raging all over the City where gas mains had been ripped apart; and then, with the noise of fire engines tearing along and ambulances hooting, the City around the hospital was bedlam.

As far as I can remember, the attack itself must have lasted only about ten or fifteen minutes, before the Zeppelin rose swiftly into the night sky, retreating silently and safely to its base in Germany. Of all the Zeppelin raids on London during the war, this one was supposedly the costliest, in monetary terms. Fortunately, the City's historic buildings and monuments were, by and large, left alone.

In January 1916, four months after this unforeseen attack on London, and having fully qualified and completed our terms as housemen, my friends and I each obtained a temporary commission in the Royal Army Medical Corps, with the rank of lieutenant.

We proceeded to buy our uniforms: sand-brown in colour, and a peaked cap with the medical badge of Aesculapius, the Greek god of medicine and healing, adorning the front. We were also given a warm woollen overcoat and a sleeping bag. Among the smaller kit items were a set of basic medical instruments, a compass, a map and whistle and a pair of folding binoculars.

Our orders were to report to the commanding officer at Tweseldown Camp near Aldershot in Surrey. Here we met several hundred other young doctors from various hospitals and we slept in tents. By day we became familiar with the RAMC's organization of medical services – a chain of evacuation – which comprised a series of routes back from the front line, via posts and stations, by which we would have to collect the sick and wounded and, if need be, transport them to base hospitals either in France or England via hospital ship. We also occupied many boring hours doing stretcher drill by numbers, and each week batches of men would leave to join various army units who were in action in France and Flanders (the Western Front), Egypt, Salonica and Africa. With some impatience, we awaited our turn.

Eventually three of us received our orders and were told we were going overseas to France and that, once at Abbeville, we should report to the Deputy Director of Medical Services (DDMS). The great day arrived when we left Waterloo by train for Southampton, thence to embark on a troopship for the French port of Le Havre. I shall never forget our journey up the River Seine to Rouen, in northern France. Scores of French children and adults were running along the banks waving Union Jacks and the brightly coloured tricolours, shouting, '*Bravo! Vive les Anglais, vive les Anglais!*'

In due course we arrived at Rouen, one of the main hospital bases for the British Expeditionary Force during the war, where we spent a few days before embarking for Abbeville. Our daily ration comprised a tin of McConaghy's meat stew – some tins were actually left over from the Boer War – army biscuits, bars of chocolate, tinned milk, and tea and sugar already mixed together in a small paper packet. The stew, in spite of its apparent age, was excellent, as was the chocolate, but the army biscuits required the attention of a chisel or bayonet!

On our arrival at Abbeville, situated on the River Somme, we reported to the DDMS, as ordered.

'You, Lieutenant,' I was told, 'will be joining Ambulance Train No. 22.'

3

'*À Bas Les Boches*'

A Doctor on Ambulance Train 22

THE AMBULANCE TRAIN was truly magnificent. It was painted a khaki colour, with a large red cross – the sign of neutrality – on a circular white background on the sides and roof. There were three medical officers to each train, as well as three nursing sisters, a Royal Army Medical Corps sergeant and about thirty-five other ranks. Our train was made up of reconverted London and North Western Railway rolling stock, which had been shipped to France the previous year. There were approximately sixteen coaches, more than half of which were ward cars, with a separate coach for infectious diseases. There was one carriage for sitting cases, while the remainder were cot cars for the more seriously wounded and bedridden patients – each car offering tiered berths for up to thirty-six patients. There was also a dining car, a kitchen and accommodation for the medical staff. All coaches had electric light and steam heating. Our train would travel up and down the line between the various casualty clearing stations, and would convey the seriously wounded to the various base hospitals, where they generally stood a better chance of survival.

Casualty clearing stations were mostly large, tented camps or a collection of huts located close to a railway line, with space for at least 200 sick and wounded at any one time. Here the medic's job was to get the injured soldier back to the front line as soon as possible – often this would mean treating the less-serious cases first. The more-serious cases were cared for until well enough to travel, but the basic accommodation and unsanitary conditions meant that casualty clearing stations were not a suitable place for long-term convalescence.

Sick men were also being treated: venereal diseases were common, as was trench foot – a crippling fungal infection of the foot caused by hours of standing in the wet and cold, and which, if not treated quickly, could turn gangrenous and result in amputation.

During the first year of the war hundreds of men were being invalided to casualty clearing stations with the label DAH, which stood for 'disordered action of the heart'. For a while medical officers were completely baffled, then at last the mystery was solved: men were removing the bullets from cartridge cases and were chewing the grains of explosive, which contained nitroglycerine. When ingested, this will drop blood pressure and cause the heart to race. When the troops heard that the medics had become wise to their tricks, this complaint disappeared almost as quickly as it had begun.

One bombardier certainly deserved better luck, for his ingenuity. One day, at one of my sick parades – where all men who were sick, or who thought they were, reported for examination and treatment – this man reported that he was unwell with a discharge from his genitals, which appeared to be pus. There was only one diagnosis: the venereal disease gonorrhoea.

'Now, Bombardier,' I said, 'I cannot treat you with this complaint in the line, so you will have to be sent down to No. 9 Hospital Le Havre, where all venereal-disease cases are treated.'

'Oh, but sir, I don't want to leave all my pals in the gun line,' he protested. 'Can't you possibly treat me?'

'Impossible,' I said, and so down the line the bombardier went.

Two weeks later I received a very stern letter from the DDMS at Le Havre concerning the bombardier and stating: this man is a lead-swinger; before reporting to you and exhibiting his discharge, he filled a fountain-pen filler with some ration Ideal milk, squirted this up his genital organ and then reported sick. His discharge was duly microscoped and revealed no gonococci, but hundreds of fat globules! He is being court-martialled immediately, and you are hereby warned to keep an eye out for similar cases.

ON AMBULANCE TRAIN 22 our runs would be quite varied, and we saw a good deal of Belgium and France on our travels. As we journeyed through the picturesque Rhône Valley during the peach harvest, barrels of peaches were loaded onto the train for the sick and wounded. As I was a non-smoker, I used to collect my issue of ration cigarettes and hand them over to the French engine drivers, who, because of this acceptable gift, allowed me to drive the engine when we were travelling empty up the line. During one run down to Marseilles I was allowed to spend several hours in the cab of one of the large PLM Express engines. The French railway lines, in those days, were in a bad state of repair, and I recall that the whole train would rock precariously as we sped along over the diamond-shaped points.

Two rail journeys in particular remain with me. In 1916 our train was the first to travel to Marseilles to collect the sick and wounded brought by sea from Salonica in northern Greece, where our troops had, for more than a year, been supporting Serbia against an invasion by Germany, Austria–Hungary and Bulgaria. The men we treated not only suffered from debilitating diseases such as malaria, typhoid and dysentery or from horribly infected wounds – all of which rendered them incapable of taking any further part in hostilities – but many were mentally affected by their experiences as well.

On another occasion our train was chosen to take some 200 German officers – again chronically sick and wounded prisoners – to Switzerland, in exchange for a similar number of British officers (also prisoners) from Germany. I shall never forget the sight of these German officers. When our train arrived at the docks with the hospital ship moored alongside, we saw them disembark resplendent in full regimental dress uniforms, which had apparently been sent to them from Germany before their departure. They looked rather like the chorus of a musical comedy – there were Uhlans, Death's Head Hussars, Prussian Guards and other elite formations, with shining pike-staffs and brilliantly coloured uniforms. Our Tommies in their shabby khaki looked a miserable lot beside these magnificent specimens; and how our medical orderlies longed to get their hands on some of the spiked German helmets as souvenirs!

As we were travelling across France on our way to the Swiss border, where the exchange was to take place, I happened to be sitting in a coach with about forty German officers. We were moving slowly through a French station when I asked my sergeant, who was accompanying me, to put his head out the window and let me know where we were. As he looked out, he was repeatedly struck by a Frenchman with a long beard, who was running alongside the train. It took the stunned sergeant a second to realize that the weapon was an umbrella.

'*À bas les Boches, à bas les Boches!*' ['Down with the Germans!'] the Frenchman shouted hysterically at him.

He apparently mistook my sergeant for a German officer, as the local inhabitants had been warned that this special train would be passing through their town. You can imagine the hilarity and merriment with which the German officers viewed this episode. They thought it a huge joke, much to the discomfort of my sergeant, who was unusually quiet for the remainder of the journey. I imagine that Frenchman told his family that evening, 'Your father has struck for France this day – I hit one of those hateful Boche on the head.'

Throughout my time on Ambulance Train 22 we carried,

and treated, wounded German personnel as well as our own Allied troops, and the futility of war was often brought home to me, especially when I saw our men playing cards and exchanging cigarettes with their erstwhile enemies. I talked to a number of Germans whose war service was finished, owing to tuberculosis or some chronic disability. Among them was one of the Zeppelin officers whose airship had been shot down over the Thames. He told me that he had previously been a clerk in a London City bank.

At this stage of the war men were dying in their thousands from gas gangrene. This was a fatal disease, caused by a germ that was driven into the flesh by a bullet or shell splinter, thereby carrying death with it. It was an anaerobe bacillus – in other words, it could only do its deadly work in the absence of air. It was called gas gangrene on account of the bubbles of gas forming under the skin. The disease, once present, advanced rapidly and the only hope in those days was amputation of the affected limb.

One captured German sergeant-major told me how he owed his life to a bluebottle fly – it was an extraordinarily interesting case. This man had been lying in a shell hole in no-man's-land, the area between the two opposing trenches, for several days and had a large, gaping wound in the middle of his right thigh, which was crawling with hundreds of maggots. Obviously, a bluebottle fly must have laid its eggs inside his wound and the little emerging maggots had, by aerating it, saved the man's life by preventing the onset of the prevalent and much-dreaded gas gangrene.

*

EVERY NOW AND THEN our train would have a general over-haul and spring-clean – on one occasion we stayed in Amiens for a weekend, where tier upon tier of sandbags surrounded the town's beautiful cathedral. And on several occasions our train evacuated the wounded from Albert, the Allies' main town behind the lines closest to the 1916 Somme battlefields. There a golden statue of the Virgin Mary and infant Jesus adorned the spire of the Albert church. It had been hit by shellfire early on in the war, and the Virgin Mary appeared to be leaning in a near-horizontal position. There was a saying that whoever made the statue fall would lose the war.

Another time we stayed at Solteville, the railway yard outside Rouen. While there, we had to use the station-yard lavatories, consisting of two rows of some half-dozen water closets. On one side *Hommes* and on the other side *Femmes*, with a partition between them, but low enough to allow one to speak to a lady friend on the other side – this was France after all!

We stopped in Rouen during the winter when the Seine froze over and, after hiring some skates, several of us skated for many miles up and down the icy river. We also played a rather ragged game of ice-hockey. We felt safe enough, though early one morning we heard an aeroplane flying low overhead. I looked out of the carriage window and, to my amazement, directly above us, saw a German Fokker plane with the black iron cross painted on its tail. The pilot was clearly visible and waved to us in a most friendly manner. He obviously noted the red cross on our train and so left us alone.

On another occasion our ambulance train spent a few days at Abbeville for an overhaul and, while there, I saw a contingent of our gallant allies – the Portuguese – arrive. I was rather amused to see their officers dressed in lavender-coloured uniforms and patent-leather boots with grey felt tops and mother-of-pearl buttons. It did not seem quite the foot-wear for muddy trenches, especially considering the many cases of trench foot that we medics were treating at the time.

The following day a goods train drew up in the station yard, with long trucks behind it on which there appeared to be tractors, covered by tarpaulins. There were a number of sentries guarding the train and we were told it carried some-thing very hush-hush. Later on we discovered that these were the first tanks to go into action shortly afterwards in the Somme, towards the end of 1916, in an attempt to help break the stalemate of trench warfare and bring some mobility back to the Western Front.

We had a wonderful RAMC cook on board our train; he could transform tins of corned beef (or 'bully beef', as it was known) into a dozen different dishes. In spite of his talent there was a certain monotony to our food, and during this time I couldn't help noticing that we generally got either plum or apple jam, and never saw kidneys or liver. I learned why from a cousin of mine, who was a major in the Army Service Corps at one of the French ports. On one occasion our train stayed here for twenty-four hours and I enjoyed a magnificent meal with him.

'It's all ration food. How do you like it?' he asked.

I could hardly believe it.

'Ah,' he said, 'our quartermaster sergeant sees that we get the strawberry jam, the sheep's kidneys and liver, and so on. Then we send the carcass up to you chaps!'

I told him exactly what I thought of him and his quartermaster!

Then, in late summer 1917, I received a message to report to the DDMS when we were next at Abbeville, and thereafter my days as an ambulance-train medical officer were numbered. Instead I was ordered to join the 59th Brigade Royal Field Artillery as their medical officer. This horse-drawn unit was one of numerous RFA brigades responsible for the medium-calibre guns and howitzers and, as the batteries were generally deployed about half a mile from the front-line trenches, I was hopeful that I would now see some actual fighting.

4

'Run Like a Stag, Sir'

A Doctor on the Western Front

MY NEW BRIGADE had just moved to the Loos area and although there were no major engagements at this time, equally there was no let-up in the day-to-day hostilities of entrenched warfare, in the usual harassing fire and in the human suffering, which my RAMC orderly and I managed to the best of our ability. We medical officers were not expected to engage in battle, and many of us chose to perform our duties unarmed. I was equipped with a medical pannier, which contained basic first-aid items such as dressings, morphia, chloroform, splints and anti-tetanus serum.

On my arrival I had discovered that my commanding officer and I had been at the same public school, so we had something in common.

'First things first,' he said. 'We should go and see where our four batteries are dug in, so that you can fix up your medical-aid posts.'

During battle these first-aid posts were generally set up quite close behind the front, so that both the walking wounded and more seriously injured soldiers would not have far to go and could be treated quickly. My CO and I were just walking over some shell-pocked ground when the German artillery suddenly put down a barrage. It was my first experience of shellfire and, on seeing my startled reaction, my CO calmly suggested that 'We should climb into a shell-hole until this noise blows over.'

'We are quite safe here, as no shell *ever* falls twice in the same shell-hole,' he said, trying his best to encourage me.

I was grateful for his reassuring remarks, though I'm not sure I was entirely convinced, and for some time I had an extremely unpleasant feeling in my stomach.

Our mess and our sleeping bunks were at the time situated in dugouts behind the remains of what was once the town of Loos. I shared sleeping bunks with three other officers – one was a mad Irishman. Each evening our batman, an army orderly, placed a large canvas bucket of water on the floor, which we used for washing in the morning. I once woke up in the middle of the night to hear a curious dik-dik-dik sound and, flashing my torch onto the floor, saw five huge rats sitting on the edge of the bucket, drinking. The light of my torch promptly woke up my Irish friend, who whipped out his revolver and fired point-blank at the bucket. The rats vanished unscathed, but a bullet penetrated the bottom of the bucket and our ablutions the following morning were scanty.

As the unsanitary conditions of the trenches worsened, so began an infestation of rats – both black and brown varieties, some of them as big as cats. I soon discovered how bold these rodents were, for I awoke one morning to find that one had gnawed its way right through my haversack, which I used as a pillow, and had all but completely demolished a bar of chocolate I kept in there. It made me shudder to think that it had enjoyed its meal a few inches from my sleeping face.

AFTER A FEW WEEKS our guns were sent to the La Bassée Canal section and I recall one glorious sunny afternoon when my bombardier batman and I set off to locate the new position of our batteries and fit up some regimental aid posts. Although these were mostly located in dugouts or deep shell-holes, on this occasion we were exploring a communication trench, which ran parallel to the main road and was used generally to enable men and materials to move to and from the firing trenches. In the distance we could see rows of German sausage-shaped observation balloons. All was peaceful, with not a shell being fired from either side. Suddenly – from out of nowhere – jumped a hare. Foolishly my bombardier and I leapt onto the road and ran after it, not that we had any chance of catching it, but for a little exercise. We were just approaching a crossroad when we heard the whining sound of a shell. At the same time I saw my batman, who had been in the retreat from Mons – the British Army's first major confrontation of the war, in August 1914 – and seemed to know all about shells, fall flat on his stomach. Following his example, I dropped to the ground, which shuddered beneath me. My batman quickly jumped up.

'Run like a stag, sir, run like a stag, sir!' he shouted at me.

I certainly did not need to be told twice. I jumped up and we raced off. We had hardly covered thirty yards when a second shell hit that crossroad and exploded with a terrific bang – the first one, miraculously for us, having been a dud.

That night in the mess dugout I told my commanding officer about our adventure.

'You bloody, bloody fools!' he yelled. 'Why on earth do you think those German observation balloons are there? Don't you know that the Boche has a gun taped on every crossroad, to blast idiots like you off the face of the Earth – and you damn well deserved it! As you ran down that road you were observed by those balloons, and the battery was phoned to fire at the very moment you reached the crossroad.'

After that little adventure I kept to the communication trench and stayed well away from the crossroads.

THAT OCTOBER OF 1917 we were told we were moving north, but before doing so we would be able to rest in billets in a deserted old French château, well behind the front line. Our brigade needed the respite because – unlike the infantry, who rested in the reserve lines or went into billets many miles behind the line – gunners in those days tended to remain for

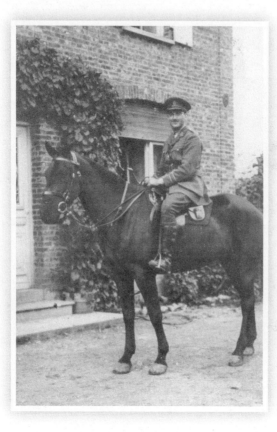

October 1917.

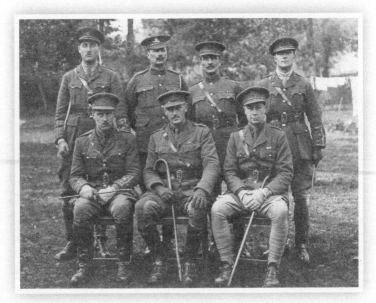

Officers of the 59th Brigade Royal Artillery, 1917.

much longer in one sector and were therefore in sustained action for a more protracted period.

I had a very fine steed at the time and used to enjoy riding through some woods nearby, scented by wild lily-of-the-valley. Sometimes I would tie my horse to a tree and, for an hour or so, would lie on my back in the long grass, listening to the birds singing. It was utterly tranquil there, and it was almost incomprehensible to think that some fifty miles away men were slaughtering one another.

In due course we arrived at a sector north of Ypres. The Battle of Passchendaele was raging all around us. As I had previously done duty in the gun line, it was now my turn to stay with the wagon line, where the horses, limbers and other vehicles were kept, along with various support elements of the brigade.

In general the wagon line was situated about a mile further back from the guns, but it was still often a target for enemy attack because, without ammunition and horses, the gunners' efficiency would be greatly affected. Here we slept in tents, though we did not get much sleep at all, as we were continuously being disturbed by a high-velocity gun from the Houthulst Forest firing at us intermittently. We would hear the loud boom of the cannon and then, a few seconds later, the shell would burst.

Behind our tents was a narrow-gauge railway line on which ammunition and other supplies were sent up each night. During the first night one of these shells landed on the tracks and a large piece of rail came hurtling down on our tent, cutting two of the ropes, so that the tent immediately collapsed and half a dozen of us officers struggled to extract ourselves from canvas and ropes in the pitch-dark. Miraculously no one was wounded, but it was a complete shambles, and at this point I rather wished I was back on the gun line.

Our wagon line was based at Vlamertinghe in West Flanders, but our guns remained due east across the Ypres–Yser canal, at a spot known as Lancashire Farm. The constant shelling and the heavy rain produced a thick mud, which hampered my daily visits to the gun line, where some of the worst injuries that I treated were those inflicted by artillery.

I would have to cross a bridge over the canal, which was observed by the German artillery, and there was a (thankfully) short period when they would put down a barrage at any time of the day or night, on sighting someone on the bridge. As a result, these crossings became increasingly hazardous, and speed was of the essence – long gone were the days when we stopped to skim stones on the river.

WE RECEIVED 125 francs a month as pay, which at the time was worth about five pounds. Some of this we would use to play bridge or poker at night. Some months I would be well in, and at other times almost bankrupt. We occasionally went into the Flemish town of Poperinge (or 'Pops', as we knew it), where an army chaplain by the name of the Rev. 'Tubby' Clayton had founded Toc H – a rest home for battle-weary soldiers, open to every man, regardless of rank. It became very well known, and there was also an excellent cafe nearby called Skindles, where you got grilled sole, roast duck and other delicacies. It was a vast improvement on army rations, and it was good to forget about the day's hardships and to socialize with officers from other units.

Like the Somme, the countryside here was nothing but mud, shell-holes, rolls upon rolls of barbed wire, wooden duckboards and battered tree stumps. It reminded me of one of the grim illustrations from *Dante's Inferno*. Due to the incessant rain, shell-holes were often filled with water that, owing to the clay soil, never drained away. Any exhausted or wounded Tommy who strayed off a duckboard and fell into a shell-hole – which often happened at night – was more than likely to drown, as there was no hold on the wet clay walls, so it was almost impossible to escape.

Later on, it was my turn to return to the gun line, where the conditions were appalling – there was water and mud every-where and we lived in waterproof boots, to avoid getting the dreaded trench foot.

My grandfather did not record specific details of the injuries he treated during the war, but he did always say that he honed his surgical skills on the Western Front. Considering that artillery experts tell us the white-hot steel shrapnel from an exploding shell – of the kind used in the First World War – travelled faster than the speed of sound, and could quite literally tear a man to pieces, one can perhaps appreciate his reticence to recall such cases.

His initial enthusiasm at being closer to the action must soon have faded, as the grim reality of life and death in the trenches (and of the limitations imposed on him in his ability to do his job) became apparent. It must have been vastly different from his many months on an ambulance train – miles from the front line – where it was altogether calmer, the conditions were more manageable and the men he examined and treated had already received some medical attention.

As well as trench foot, there were other virulent trench-borne diseases that caused great misery and suffering among the troops at this time: trench fever, with its achy flu-like symptoms trans-mitted by body lice; and trench mouth, which was a painful ulcerating mouth condition caused by stress, smoking and a poor diet and oral hygiene – all unavoidable elements of life in the dugouts on the Western Front.

There were also the men who staggered to the aid posts after gas attacks; blistered and blinded, they were nevertheless con-sidered fortunate survivors. Some men were mentally broken, displaying the telltale signs of shell-shock: a distant stare and the inability to speak.

Add to these very real medical scenarios the constant threat of death as you carried out your work, the makeshift surgeries amid the glutinous, filthy mud and the hordes of rats made fat on the ready supply of corpses, and one can see what a desperate struggle it must have been for my grandfather and other RAMC officers like him to keep men alive and sufficiently well to continue fighting.

BY APRIL 1918, after two years on the Western Front, I was the only survivor of our original Barts quintet who had joined the army as medical officers; two of my friends were killed at

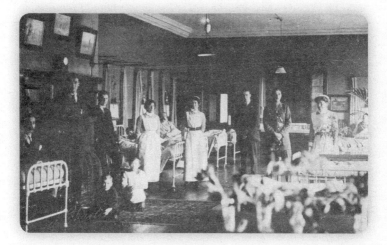

South African Military Hospital in Richmond Park, 1918.

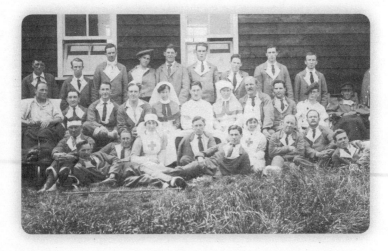

Some of my patients and the sisters of Good Hope ward, June 1918.

Gallipoli in the Dardanelles campaign, and the other two in France. At this time my own health had begun to suffer as I developed a duodenal ulcer – aggravated by life on the front and not improved by a daily diet of bully beef and stale biscuits – so I put in for a transfer back to England, where I could continue my duties and receive medical treatment for my own condition.

I was duly transferred back to London and joined the staff of the newly built South African Hospital in Richmond Park, which had been financed by wealthy South Africans under the chairmanship of Lord Gladstone, to accommodate wounded South African troops during the war. Soon after I joined, a further demand for beds resulted in the hospital being merged with the Richmond Military Hospital and renamed the South African Military Hospital, whereupon I was placed in charge of two of the large surgical wards, with about ninety patients in each.

Being back in England made it easier to renew my friendship with Rosamund Nancy Tracey, the cousin of my old school friend Alex Sim. We had kept in touch during the war and, now that I was based in London, we were able to spend some time together. Since the carefree school holidays we had spent together as youngsters in Devon, Nan – as she was now known to me – had grown into a charming young woman. She was also extremely well read, especially in the classics, and I always enjoyed it when she would recite Shakespeare and other prose to me. She also spoke fluent French. Sometimes, on one of my rare evenings off duty, we would go to the West End to see a show or to a piano recital as we both adored classical music. In the months that followed, our affection for one another deepened and she made me very happy when she accepted my proposal of marriage. We decided to hold the ceremony at the ancient church of St Saviour's in Dartmouth, Devon, where her father had once been vicar.

It so happened that one of my patients at Richmond at the time was also a man in love, who was prepared to make a rather drastic sacrifice for his fiancée. He had recently been admitted as a casualty from France with several pieces of shrapnel in his chest, which had to be removed. Despite his serious wounds he was able to move about with little discomfort and, as such, was one of the patients who was allowed to take light exercise in Richmond Park.

Apparently on one of these walks he got friendly with a local Richmond girl, romance blossomed and he proposed to her. The patient must have had native South African heritage, for although his skin was moderately light in colour, he had a classic native nose. His friend agreed to marry him, but only on condition that he had an operation on his nose – to rectify its broad flatness. I mentioned this to the chief surgeon, who seemed quite content to help this love affair along. So while our patient was on the operating table, incisions were made around the flat nostrils and an aperture was created at the point of the nose. An instrument was pushed up through this aperture and was moved from side to side to separate the skin from the underlying tissues. After this, with the patient's prior permission, the cartilage of one of his ribs was removed, suitably shaped and then inserted and pushed up through the hole and moulded into place. The side-flaps of the nostrils were brought towards the centre and stitched, as was the aperture through which the cartilage was finally inserted. The shrapnel was then removed from his chest.

Some six weeks later our corporal was discharged with a handsome new aquiline nose. We never heard of him again, and hoped that his fiancée did not let him down and that the marriage duly took place.

At the end of hostilities on 11 November 1918, jubilant crowds gathered outside Buckingham Palace and in Trafalgar Square, and in public spaces all over London, to celebrate the signing of the Armistice.

Two weeks later, on 27 November 1918, Nan and I were married. Friends and family gathered to wish us well and I was particularly pleased to see my two brothers, Rupert and Denis, as I had not seen them since before we had left to take up our various roles in the Great War. Here we were, three brothers together once more – fortunate survivors! Denis had been a cadet in the artillery, and Rupert, who was older, had served with the 22nd Manchester Regiment. He proudly showed us his Military Cross war medal, Britain's third-highest military decoration for valour, which he had been awarded for his part in an attack on Munich Trench near Serre in France in 1917. We were all very impressed, especially when a year or so later he was honoured once again, this time with the Al Valore Militare, the Italian equivalent of the Victoria Cross, for his role in the 1918 Battle of the River Piave.

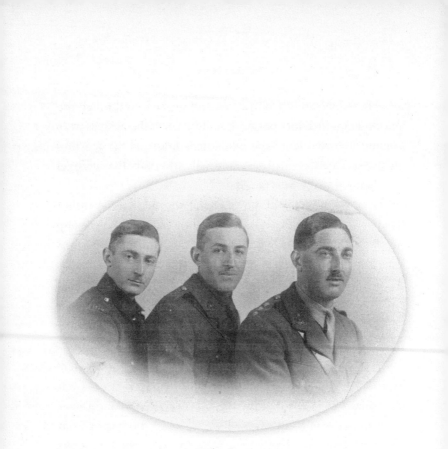

Denis, Rupert and me, 1918.

Our father had travelled from South Africa especially for the wedding and, as it happens, was also happily reunited with our mother, who had been living in London for much of the war, to be closer to Rupert and me, should one of us fall ill or be wounded while we were posted abroad.

There was a sombre moment during the marriage ceremony itself when the congregation members were asked to pray for fallen brothers. Nan's only brother, a cadet in what was then called the Royal Flying Corps, had been just eighteen years old when he had been killed in a training exercise accident in May 1918. Later on his name – Ernest Osborne Tracey – was included on a wooden plaque that hangs in St Saviour's, honouring all those parish members who lost their lives during the Great War.

AFTER WE WERE MARRIED Nan and I went to live in a small flat off the Edgware Road, which we shared with Rupert, who had resumed his architectural studies in London. One day we were chatting and he told me a rather curious story concerning another member of our family. Rupert had been walking up Regent Street when he met a brother officer to whom he had lent a small sum of money. This officer had forgotten to repay the loan and felt very embarrassed on accidentally meeting my brother.

'Look here, old man,' Rupert's friend said, 'I am still rather hard up, but I have an old Chinese ornament in my flat, and you are welcome to have this, to square the deal.'

He was most insistent, and so my brother went to his flat

and acquired the ornament. A short while later he took it to the Ceramic Department at the British Museum and was told that it was some 300 years old and very valuable. A curator described the period in which it was made, but was unable to value it. Not being particularly interested in antiques, my brother advertised it in the personal column of *The Times* under a box number. He received only one reply and, strangely enough, it was from one of our uncles, who had spent many years in Shanghai and collected this particular kind of china.

There was another bizarre coincidence concerning the same uncle when I was a patient at the New Lodge Clinic in Windsor Park some time later. I was enduring various tests for the duodenal ulcer I had developed during the war – one of the most unpleasant being the passing of a long tube into the stomach for what is known as a barium-meal test. The nurse who was administering this torture for the purpose of an X-ray said, 'Cheer up. I passed a similar tube on a patient we had here a few years ago, and this patient saw the funny side of it and, being a good cartoonist, said to me: "When I am eventually allowed up, I will draw a series of cartoons for you."'

True to his word, the cartoons were drawn, and the clinic's management liked them and therefore framed and hung them around the walls of the dining room.

One of the cartoons showed a man balancing a stomach-tube on the end of his nose and was reminiscent of John Tenniel's drawing of Old Father William in *Alice's Adventures in Wonderland*. All the drawings were signed and the artist, of all people, was none other than the same uncle who had written to my brother enquiring about the Chinese ornament. Unbeknown to me, he had also been a patient at this clinic some years previously.

Although the war had ended in 1918, I wasn't officially discharged from my duties at Richmond Park until July the following year, whereupon I managed to secure a standard six-month term as house surgeon at the Hospital for Sick Children in Great Ormond Street – the country's first-ever specialist hospital for all child-related medical matters, which had been founded in 1852.

Testimonials

South African Military Hospital
Richmond Park
Surrey

25 June 1919

Captain White-Cooper has worked in the surgical division of this hospital for the past 12 months. He is in every way a satisfactory medical officer. I found him highly efficient, careful and tactful in his treatment of the patients. He has performed many operations and can also be considered an experienced surgical clinician. I have pleasure in giving him this testimonial and can confidently recommend him for any surgical position for which he may apply.

Thomas Lindsay Sandes
Lt Col, Surgical Division

South African Military Hospital
Richmond Park
Surrey

9 July 1919

This is to certify that Captain W. R. White-Cooper joined the RAMC in January 1916 and transferred to the South African Medical Corps in April 1918 after serving two years in France. Since April 1918 he has had charge of two large surgical wards (averaging 90 patients) in this hospital. Captain White-Cooper has done his work here very well indeed and his wards have been administered to my entire satisfaction. He is a painstaking officer – a good surgeon and a pleasant colleague – and I have much pleasure in strongly recommending him as a House Surgeon for the Hospital for Sick Children Great Ormond Street.

Colonel Edward Thornton
Hospital Commandant

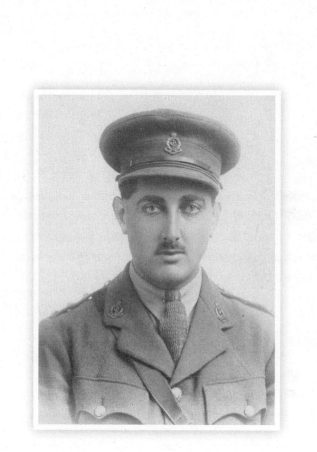

July 1919.

'My late husband was brought into the world by your grandfather in 1920. In fact, he claimed to be the first baby Dr White-Cooper ever delivered in Dartmouth! Both he and his mother swore by your grandfather, and no doctor that followed him ever compared. We lived in Albert Place and they were very happy times.'

YVONNE LEGG, 2012

5

'Us Likes a Nice Bottle of Medicine'

A New GP in Devon

IN MARCH 1920, on completion of my term at the Hospital for Sick Children, Nan and I decided to move to Devon, where I could continue my career as a GP. Nan was expecting our first child and so it made perfect sense for us to settle in Dartmouth, where she herself had been born and where her mother, Alice Tracey, known to the family as 'Cubby', still lived. Of course we also had very fond memories of many happy school holidays spent together at her cousin's home in nearby Brixham.

Dartmouth is a naval port with a rich history, set in a quiet, picturesque location on the River Dart. The town had several ship-building businesses, which were not as busy then as they had been before the war; and steamers would still stop to take on coal, though increasingly oil-burning engines were becoming more common. On a fine day the rolling South

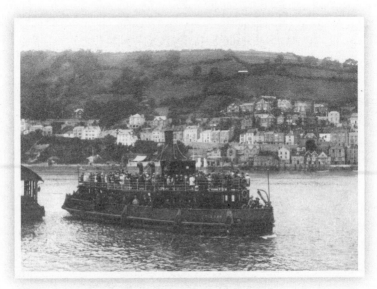

A ferry crossing the River Dart, Dartmouth, 1919.

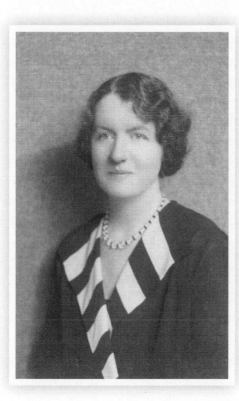

My wife, Nan.

Hams countryside, which surrounds the town, resembles a giant patchwork quilt, and I was very pleased to be living in such a scenic town and to have left city life behind me. For the first year we based ourselves with Cubby, at the family home of North Ford House in North Ford Road, an attractive Regency-style villa situated in a narrow, winding lane above the market in the town centre.

The layout of North Ford House was such that we kept our trap inside a garage downstairs (at this time I travelled everywhere in a horse and trap) and, from there, a few steps up led to a waiting room, with chairs against the walls. My surgery lay beyond this with a small dispensary attached, where I would make up all my prescriptions at the end of each day. We lived upstairs. Nan was a very keen gardener, and all year round the veranda at the front of the house was attractively decorated with flowers in hanging baskets, which my patients always admired.

I had a brass plaque engraved with my credentials for the front entrance, and simply hoped that patients would come. Nan's family was well connected and respected locally, which greatly helped. In those days doctors would have both private and 'panel' patients – the latter being part of a health-insurance scheme established in 1911, where those below a certain income and their employers would share a flat-rate contribution to the scheme, and in return receive free but limited care from a doctor on a local list or panel. Doctors would also receive a standard payment for each panel patient they treated. This was of course long before the National Health Service existed.

I also performed operations at the nearby Dartmouth & Kingswear Hospital, a purpose-built hospital located on the town's South Embankment overlooking the river, which had replaced the original cottage hospital in Bayard's Cove back in the early 1890s. It had two main wards, with six beds in each, and an operating theatre. I believe that in the old hospital all surgical procedures took place in the wards themselves – in full view of other patients!

At North Ford House there were designated surgery times each morning and evening, and during the afternoon I would make house calls to patients in outlying villages such as Strete, Stoke Fleming, Dittisham and Blackawton. As many people did not have telephones in those early days, they would leave written messages at their local village post office for me to visit them. I would then either telephone the various post offices or stop by in person to see if I was needed – unless, of course, it was an emergency, and then my surgery would be contacted immediately.

As spring turned to summer I felt sure that I had made the right decision to become a General Practitioner. During consulting hours at one's surgery one never knows who or what the next appointment will bring, and it is this constant variety that makes the work of a GP so interesting. Personally I would not care to be a specialist, seeing so many cases of a similar nature every day. I have had children with beads stuck up their noses, small stones in the ear and fish-hooks in the hand. However, the following case was quite unusual.

One morning a little boy was brought into the surgery with

a china chamber pot crowning his head. Normally a cheerful, mischievous young lad, he was by now looking rather subdued and even tearful. His mother was clearly unamused at the time. As the chamber pot had been pushed down over his ears, it was impossible to remove it without tearing the ear, so we took him to hospital, where he was anaesthetized. Using a small hammer, I carefully cracked the chamber pot and, piece-by-piece, the broken china was delicately removed. The boy skipped off, none the worse for his ordeal.

Today the old-fashioned china chamber pot is almost a museum piece, but that was not so when I first started in practice. On two occasions my patients were stout ladies who had sat down on them so heavily that the chamber broke under them, in each case causing deep lacerations of the buttocks. These were rapidly sutured and healed satisfactorily. Fortunately this is an accident that has disappeared for good since the modern plastic toilet seat came into universal use.

By now I was also starting to gain patients in the town's outlying villages, where I began to hold regular surgeries. These were real Devonshire country folk, some of whom were totally illiterate, but nonetheless delightful people. However, it soon became apparent that one or two of them were more than a little wary of me, and would clearly take some time to get used to me – and my ways.

One day a new patient of mine, a farmer, decided to confide in me.

'Doc, you will have to make some changes, if you wish to build a successful practice amongst the locals,' he said.

'What do you mean?'

'Well, I overheard this conversation in the local public house the other night. There were two men talking, and one said, "'Ere, what do you think of this young doc wot's 'ere?" His friend said, "Us don't think much of him. He sent us out some little sweeties – but us likes a nice bottle of medicine wot us has to shake."'

On hearing this, I made a mental note to make sure that no more tablets were sent to that particular village.

WE WERE VERY FORTUNATE that people in Dartmouth were so welcoming. Nan and I were invited to a local dance, where I was to be officially introduced as the new doctor in town. I was at home, getting dressed up in my dinner jacket and black tie, and we were just about to leave the house when the telephone rang. As I lifted the receiver I heard piercing yells and shouts, which almost obscured the voice of the hospital matron.

'Oh, Doctor, please come at once,' she pleaded. 'I have a man here rolling around on the bed, shouting and yelling, and we cannot control him.'

'What's his story?' I asked.

'Well, he says that half an hour ago he went to the toilet and since then he has been in agony in his rectal region.'

I drove down to the hospital and as soon as the patient saw me he screamed, 'For God's sake, Doctor, help me! I feel as if I have a dagger in my backside.'

I asked the matron for a sterile rubber glove, well Vaselined, told the patient to lie on his side and slowly inserted my index finger into his rectum. Within an inch of the orifice I came across a hard object, similar to a matchstick, lying across the rectal wall.

'Tell me, sir, have you been sticking matches up your rectum?' I asked.

'Certainly not!' said the man. 'But for God's sake – whatever it is – get it out.'

'Well,' I replied, 'I might hurt you a little more, but get it out I will.'

Using a plug of cotton wool soaked in a local anaesthetic solution, I treated the rectum and, with some difficulty, the offending object was removed. Lo and behold, what emerged looked like a piece of a bird's rib just over an inch long.

'However did that get there?' I asked.

'Good Lord,' said my patient. 'I remember now that I had some rather good pigeon pie in Exeter, about a month ago. I recall that I swallowed something quite hard, but at the time I thought it was just a piece of pie crust.'

The interesting thing about this case was that this sharp piece of bone had taken a month to reach the rectum, without perforating the bowel at any point on its journey. Had it done so, my patient might have developed a fatal case of peritonitis – inflammation of tissues that line the inside of the abdomen. Instead, he left the hospital much relieved, and my wife and I thoroughly enjoyed the dance, in spite of arriving late.

ON 7 SEPTEMBER 1920, in our home upstairs at North Ford House, Nan was safely delivered of our first child, a son –

Michael Osborn – who weighed in at over twelve pounds. It soon became apparent that we needed more room and so, along with Cubby, we decided to move to a larger property in the town; we purchased a three-storeyed terraced Regency house, which we named 'Montagu', just five minutes' walk away in Ridge Hill. The rooms were large with high ceilings and on the ground floor there were floor-to-ceiling sash windows. There was a wonderful terrace with a cast-iron balustrade balcony at the rear that looked out over a sizeable garden, which ran all the way down to Clarence Street.

At the bottom of Ridge Hill was a public house called the Ship in Dock Inn, which was frequented each evening by workers from the local shipyard. I seem to have had a number of patients who owned public houses – not that I was a good customer; in fact, being almost teetotal, I never helped to swell their coffers. One particular publican and his wife had twenty children. He was very keen on cricket, and each year his wife would pick ten children and he a similar number, and there would be a family eleven-a-side match on the village green.

Another landlord, a ginger-haired fellow called 'Ted' by all and sundry, was an epileptic. Whenever Ted had a fit, he dislocated his jaw – in fact, people used to joke that his jaw became so loose on account of his magnificent vocabulary of swear words. Well, none of his customers or his wife Millie could put Ted's jaw back after a fit, so I would get an urgent message to come at once and reduce Ted's jaw. Having done this on about half a dozen occasions, I got rather tired of this game, so I said to Millie, 'I am going to teach you how to put your husband's jaw back.'

'Oh, I couldn't possibly do that!' she protested.

'It's really quite simple,' I replied. 'The first thing you do is get a couple of stout corks and put one on each side of his mouth between the upper and lower jaw. If you don't do this, he could bite off your fingers when his jaw snaps back into position. Then, once you have done this, and using both hands, push the lower jaw downwards and then quickly back, where-upon the jaw will slip back into its socket.'

Millie eventually had so much practice in the art of reducing a lower-jaw dislocation that I would say that, after a few months, she was perhaps England's greatest expert in this particular manoeuvre.

AFTER MOVING TO Ridge Hill we kept North Ford House as my surgery and were fortunate enough to find a retired police constable from Exeter and his family to live there as caretakers. Mr Densham was a very good handyman and his wife, whom we fondly nicknamed 'Denchie', would act as my receptionist, answering the telephone and making surgery appointments. They had a son called Tommy, who was a delightful boy.

Because our new house was built on three levels, it was not always easy to hear the front-door bell. Eventually I had an extension to my bedroom installed, so that I could hear it, but prior to this, one morning at about 1 a.m., Nan woke me to say that she had heard the night bell, so I would have to get up. I put on a dressing gown and went to the front door. On opening it, I saw a stranger aged about thirty-five, who was very apologetic at waking me at such an early hour.

'Doctor, my wife is seriously ill,' he said earnestly. 'She is vomiting and has a severe headache. Will you please come and see her?'

'All right,' I said, 'where do you live?'

'Near Totnes,' he replied, which was about eight miles away in the countryside.

'Well,' I said, 'please wait here in the hall and look at this illustrated paper, while I quickly get dressed and collect my bag.'

As we drove to his home, my travelling companion was very chatty and did not appear to be unduly perturbed about his wife's health. In fact we discussed almost every topic under the sun, except her illness.

'By the way, Doctor, what is your fee?' asked the stranger.

'Oh, don't worry, there is no need for you to settle up now,' I said, 'because I shall probably have to visit your wife again, and you can pay me when her treatment is concluded and she is well again.'

'No, Doc, I really must insist on paying you now and in cash. I always pay cash for everything I buy or do.'

'Well, if you insist,' I said, 'then a night call is a double fee, and of course there is the mileage.' The stranger paid up there and then.

As we drove into the village he pointed ahead and said, 'Doc, you see that double-storeyed house down on the left, well, that's where we live.'

So I stopped at the front of the house, whereupon the stranger hastily jumped out, eager – as I thought – to see how his poor wife was. I paused to gather my stethoscope and medical bag from the rear of the car. As I approached the front door, a light suddenly shone in an upper window and my fellow traveller stuck his head out.

'Thanks, Doc, old man,' he said cheerfully. 'I couldn't get a taxi, see. But you've had your money, and I am home – so we are both happy, aren't we? There is no one ill here. In fact I have never married.'

As you can imagine, I was not at all happy and replied, 'If you would like to come down here, I'll knock your blinkety-blinkety head off, and then there *will* be a good reason for me to treat you medically!'

Unfortunately, being called upon at all hours and in all weather was a regular feature of a doctor's life. During my first exceptionally cold and icy winter in Devon two particular visits to the countryside stayed with me. The first was to attend the birth of a very premature baby. It was at an unearthly hour that I set out in my horse and trap. There was a biting wind and the winding country lanes were still relatively new to me, so I had to drive with great care on account of the treacherous conditions. I was extremely relieved when I finally reached my patient. Both she and her husband were understandably anxious, but I managed to calm them, and the delivery itself was quite normal in all respects. As there was no crib, we made a tiny bed in a soup bowl lined with warmed cotton wraps and, mercifully, the child survived. In those days this was no mean feat.

The second incident involved a rather strange call that came at 1 a.m. one cold January morning. There had been a snowfall the previous day, so once again the roads were particularly icy. The telephone rang.

'Hello,' I said.

''Ere, is that the doctor?' asked a voice.

'Yes,' I replied.

''Ere, us wants you – to come out, see!' said the voice.

'Who is this speaking, and where do you live?' I asked.

''Ere, our Liza's dead, see – us wants you to come out.'

'Now look here,' I responded, 'if your Liza's dead, all the doctors in the world could not bring her back to life, so there is no point in my coming, is there?'

'Ah, but us ain't quite sure, see, and us be scared,' said the voice.

The village was some six miles away, but of course, as I was trying to establish myself in the area, I had to go – even though Liza wasn't my patient. As expected, I found dear Liza stone-cold dead.

'I'm afraid I can't issue a death certificate, as she was not under my care,' I told her family.

Subsequently the coroner ordered a post-mortem, which was successfully conducted, and death was found to be by natural causes. This is just an example of what doctors have to put up with. It's all in a day's – or a night's – work.

In fact, during my years as a GP in Devon, I sometimes acted for the Dartmouth police and local coroner. In the case of a drowning in the River Dart, or a death by misadventure or suicide, I would generally be asked to perform an examination or post-mortem in order to determine the cause of death. On occasion I was asked to appear as a court witness – to confirm medical facts or offer my professional opinion. I recall one appalling case when a young mother went on trial for the murder of her two young children. She had not been my patient until just before the murders, when her husband had – in desperation – arranged for me to see her, due to her feeling depressed and suffering from insomnia. She was by all accounts a good wife and a devoted mother, but must have suffered a complete and unforeseen mental breakdown. The outcome was a terrible tragedy for all concerned, and thankfully I have never again encountered a similar case. (I should add that these were the days long before antidepressants and talking therapies, when the diagnosis and medical care of those with severe depression was largely inadequate and the limited treatments available such as surgical lobotomies and electroconvulsive therapy were considered ineffectual and dangerous.)

Another dreadfully sad case that I had to deal with, when I was still quite new to Dartmouth, involved an elderly man who, having lost his wife and being stone-deaf, had come to Devon to live with his son and daughter-in-law. However, things were not working out well, and he had not been there long when I received an urgent call from the police, requesting that I visit him. I had found him lying quietly on his bed with blood pouring out from two cut wrists. The wrists were sutured and he recovered.

After that he took an overdose of sleeping tablets, but not enough to kill himself, and again he recovered. Within a month the old man had cut his throat, but once again I was able to reach him in time and save his life.

By now there was talk in the town that the daughter-in-law completely neglected the old man and half-starved him. Whatever the truth, two weeks later he jumped in front of a train, and that was the end of this likeable, poor old deaf man, who intended – no matter what the medical profession could do – to end his life of misery.

I was also once asked to perform the post-mortem on what at first sight appeared to be a readily explicable death, this time in one of Dartmouth's many boarding houses. 'Please come at once, Doctor, we have just found our lodger dead on the floor beside his bed!' was the call I received from the landlady.

Sure enough, when I got to her house the lodger was indeed dead. He was deeply cyanosed, and rigor mortis had already set in, so he must have been dead for some hours. I had never seen the man before, and as his landlady explained that he had suffered from a weak heart, I assumed his death was probably caused by a heart attack. However, as he was not a patient of mine, I was unable to give a death certificate, and later on the coroner requested that I perform a post-mortem. His heart appeared normal, his lungs deeply congested, but he had no cerebral haemorrhage or clot. I was mystified as to the cause of his death but, recalling the blue-black colour of his face, I thought I had better open up his larynx. There, wedged between his vocal cords, was a small denture that he must have dislodged in his sleep. It was unable to pass down his gullet, and so was sucked into his larynx and caused a complete blockage of air, resulting in death by suffocation.

Bizarrely, a few years later I had another patient – a naval pensioner – who suffered precisely the same fate. His wife came home and found him dead: he was in an upright position on the settee, with one set of dentures lying on the floor. During the post-mortem I recovered the top set of his dentures from his larynx. His wife explained that he had not been well at the time, so he must have been sick and put his fingers into his throat, accidentally pushing his dentures downwards, where they lodged in the throat. At the inquiry I was called as a witness, whereupon the coroner returned a verdict of death by misadventure.

As my practice became busier, I rarely managed a day off, although I did try to play a game of tennis every Wednesday afternoon. Sometimes I would take Nan on an outing to Shapley & Sons Grocers in Torquay, where she liked to buy a large wedge of Brie from France, some freshly roasted coffee beans and all manner of things that were not readily available in Dartmouth. When Michael was a little older, we would often take him for a family beach picnic at Slapton or Blackpool Sands. These excursions, however, did not always turn out successfully, as often I would be called to check on patients in villages and hamlets along the way, in which case Nan (and sometimes Michael) would have to wait patiently for many hours. I recall on one occasion that I promised to take Nan shopping for some stockings, but by the time I had done my rounds and we had driven to the stocking shop, it had long since closed and we were forced to return home empty-handed – needless to say, she was not best pleased!

We did manage a fortnight's holiday that summer, and so I hired my first locum to take care of the practice. He was a rubicund Irishman with a purplish-crimson hue to his countenance and rather shaky hands. That *should* have warned me of his weakness. Although he appeared to get through the day fairly well, when I reviewed his handwritten notes on patients at evening surgery, they were so shaky and disjointed I surmised that by then he'd had frequent nips at the bottle during the afternoon. However, he did not lose any patients; in fact, many were highly amused by his jocular manner.

With the amount of travelling I was soon required to do it seemed sensible to buy a motor car, which in the early 1920s was still a relatively uncommon sight on the country roads. The first motor car I ever owned was a maroon-coloured open Morris Oxford. I was not always the most considerate motorist. Occasionally, when I was in a hurry to attend a patient, I would leave my car kerbside; and, on more than one occasion, a sympathetic village bobby would park it for me, leaving a note on the front seat. There was very little danger of theft as most people knew my car, but I did have one interesting experience.

I had just been out to a confinement case in one of the neighbouring villages. On leaving, I placed my black maternity bag on the back seat of my car. When I got home it was dark. The next morning I got called to another confinement and, without looking in the back of the car, drove to see my patient. I returned to the car to collect my bag, but it had disappeared. Thinking I must have left it at my last patient's home, I called there, but they had not seen it. Neither was it at my home or at my surgery. I was mystified. In the meantime a medic friend lent me his bag and I was able to attend to the case. I thought: surely no one would want to steal a doctor's maternity bag? As a last resort, I decided to notify the police.

Some weeks later I realized what an amazing job the police had done, and the great trouble they had taken in tracing the bag, which as it turned out had been stolen after all. They telephoned me to say they had found the bag, but that it was in Port Talbot in Wales!

This was the story: two sailors had walked past my car and spied the bag on the back seat. One of them had lifted it and given it a good shake and, on hearing my instruments rattle, said to his friend, 'This sounds like jewellery – let's pinch it!' So they did. The next day their cargo vessel sailed from Dartmouth for Dieppe, but in the meantime they prised open the bag and, finding only doctor's instruments, one sailor suggested that they throw the bag overboard.

'No, don't do that,' his friend replied, 'there are morphia tablets in there, and we may be able to sell them to a French chemist.'

In any case they decided the instruments were of some value, so the bag was saved from the sea.

In the meantime the police searched every lodging house in the town and telephoned every police station in the county, giving a detailed description of the bag and its contents. Finally they made a note of every ship that was moored in the harbour, its date of sailing and its destination. When this particular ship left Dieppe, it sailed to Port Talbot in Wales and, on arrival, two policemen went aboard – and there, under one of the firemen's bunks, was my maternity bag.

As you can imagine, I suitably rewarded the policemen responsible, and this case just goes to show the marvellous and meticulous work carried out by Devon's police in locating an ordinary doctor's maternity bag.

Writing of maternity matters, I feel I must include an early case I had, which proved so unusual and rare that I was persuaded to go to London and describe it at one of the meetings of the Royal Society of Medicine. I had just attended a confinement case that concerned the patient's third child. The child was delivered safely with the aid of forceps, and the delivery of the afterbirth was normal in all respects. Afterwards the woman's perineum, which had been torn back to the rectum, was sutured. Over the next two weeks I visited the patient daily, as she was very anaemic, but when I came to remove the sutures, the wound gaped and seemed to show no sign of healing. I also noted that my patient seemed anxious and did not look at all well. I was just washing my hands before my examination when she suddenly sneezed several times.

'Oh, Doctor, I think perhaps I have twins, as there is a big lump between my thighs,' she exclaimed, very alarmed.

Quickly pulling back the bedclothes, I saw to my absolute astonishment that she appeared to have sneezed her womb inside out. In other words, she had what is medically known as an 'acute inversion of the uterus'. This condition, when it has been recorded, is generally due to pulling of the placenta before it has separated from the womb. I had never seen or heard of a sneeze producing it.

I immediately phoned for a colleague, who came and anaesthetized the patient, and, having douched the raw area with an antiseptic solution, we were able – with some difficulty – to return the womb to its normal position. Over the course of the next three months the patient made a full recovery and resumed her work as a village schoolteacher.

During the interwar years, women generally had their babies at home and hospital births were quite rare, except in complicated cases. This next case was certainly complex, but not in a medical sense.

Ruth was a quiet, reserved young woman of twenty-three. She lived at home with her widowed mother and helped her with dressmaking, their sole livelihood. Ruth had suffered two mild attacks of appendicitis, which had fortunately responded to medical treatment. However, I told mother and daughter that if Ruth had a third attack, I would advise surgical removal of the offending organ.

It so happened one morning, while I was operating at the hospital, that Ruth's mother telephoned to say that Ruth had had another attack of appendicitis and that this one seemed to be much more painful than the two previous ones. I told the nurse to tell Ruth's mother that I could not visit her as I was operating, but that I would send the ambulance for Ruth and that we would operate on her during the course of the morning.

The patient duly arrived at the hospital, and in the midst of the operation that we were performing a harried nursing sister opened the door to the theatre, exclaiming, 'Doctor, I believe your patient is having a baby! She has a large abdominal swelling and is having frequent pains, which suggest she is in labour.'

My assistant stitched up the skin flaps of the hernia case on which we had just operated and I hurried down to the ward, just in time to see the head of an infant emerging. Ruth's labour was normal and both she and the baby were flourishing, but her mother had a small heart attack on hearing the news, and I had to get her admitted to hospital as well. Ruth's mother had never found out about Ruth's condition and could hardly believe it.

Both mother and daughter – and grandchild – were soon well and were discharged from hospital. However, I do wonder if Ruth still has her appendix?

'We lived on a farm in the centre of Stoke Fleming, in a place known as Darkhole. I was brought into the world by your grandfather in 1927 and he also delivered my brother and sister. He would come and see us out at the farm, and whenever he appeared I knew something was up. I dreaded having injections, and he would often have to put my head through his knees in order to keep me still. He was very kind, though, and when I was older and shared with him an interest in stamp-collecting we would swap stamps. Only went he left to go back to Africa did I give him a really special one! I continued to write to him after he left and he sometimes sent me stamps.'

PHILIPPA POOK, 2012

6

'Doctor, That House Is Haunted'

Not Everything Can Be Explained

Although I felt that I had found my feet as a GP, and the practice was flourishing, I still had a lot to learn, as one of my new patients was about to show me. Betty Thompson and her parents lived in a quiet village not far from Dartmouth. They were a poor family; the father was a farm labourer and the mother took in washing. One fine autumn day I was summoned to the house, where I observed a rather pale and anaemic-looking girl lying in bed, propped up with several pillows. I was told that she had been in bed for some three years, without the strength to move, and that no doctor appeared able to help. I, as a young doctor more recently qualified and up-to-date, could surely get Betty on her feet again?

She was about twenty years old when I took over the case,

quietly spoken and gentle, with a rather sweet smile. I thought she looked so pathetic lying there in bed. Of course three years of lying in a bedroom that saw little sun had blanched her, so that she resembled a plant that had been kept under a flower pot for some weeks. I was determined to do what I could to help.

On reviewing her medical history with her mother, I gathered that one particular symptom had puzzled all previous doctors: the periodic vomiting and coughing up of blood. Her anaemia, apart from having been caused by being shut up in a small bedroom, was the natural result of blood loss. I gave Betty a thorough overhaul and, beyond a slight murmur in her heart, I could find no trace of physical disease – her lungs and abdomen appeared normal, though her reflexes were exaggerated, especially the knee jerk.

'I think most of her condition is due to nerves,' I told her mother, reassuringly.

'But, Doctor,' she said immediately, 'remember how often she has brought up blood. Surely that can't be nerves?'

'How right you are, Mrs Thompson,' I agreed.

The next morning I received an early request to visit Betty as soon as possible. When I entered the bedroom she was looking more prostrate than ever, lying flat on her back, her pillows having been removed. Under the bed was a large bowl of blood.

'Now, Doctor, come and have a look at what the poor darling has brought up this morning,' said the mother.

I agreed that it did look bad, and there was no doubt Betty was feeling much weaker for the loss.

'Well, Mrs Thompson, there is only one thing to do,' I said. 'We must admit Betty into hospital, where we can X-ray her chest and do a barium-meal test. The blood is either coming from her lungs or stomach, but I favour the former, as it does not appear like "coffee grounds", which is the usual appearance of vomited blood.'

Betty remained in hospital for some three weeks. She had no haemorrhage, all her X-rays were clear and a barium-meal test revealed no lesion. I was completely baffled, and so she returned home. I paid her visits now and then, but she certainly did not require daily visits – nor could her parents have afforded them. However, from time to time I would receive an emergency call from Mrs Thompson and there, under her daughter's bed, would be a bowl of blood. It was almost as if she timed these episodes to keep me interested, and yet there was never any physical cause that I could discover. It was a complete mystery, although I continued to believe that nerves were to blame. However, I had realized during my first visit that to mention as much to her doting mother was a major faux pas.

In fact I had recently seen another demonstration of how the mind could influence the body. It has always been recognized that there is a certain neurotic element in most asthma cases, and it was about to be proved to me that suggestion can often precipitate an attack.

A wealthy patient of mine who suffered badly from asthma insisted that flowers, especially geraniums, could initiate an attack. She also avoided cats and certain foods. When she told me that she wished to see an asthma specialist in London, I duly arranged an appointment for her and, in my report to the specialist, I mentioned her phobias. Unbeknown to my patient and to me, the specialist arranged to have a pot of artificial geraniums sent to his consulting rooms. This pot was placed on a table beside the examination couch and behind a screen. My patient and the specialist had a pleasant talk and then the specialist said, 'If you would please go behind the screen with my nurse, I would like to examine your chest.'

However, no sooner had my patient spotted the geraniums than she protested, 'Oh, my goodness, I can't breathe! Please take those dreadful flowers away.'

Within a few minutes she had produced a typical asthmatic attack. The specialist was quickly able to allay her fears and told her that the flowers were in fact artificial. He went on to explain that this proved that she associated real geranium flowers with asthma, because as soon as she had seen the pot, she had reacted as if the flowers were genuine.

I am afraid I was not in her good books when she asked me if I had told the specialist about the geraniums, and I had to confess that I had. However, we were good friends and she forgave me, and subsequently experienced no further attacks when confronted with geraniums – or any other flowers.

I have heard that an attack of asthma can be produced by certain foods, but it has not been my experience to treat such a case.

ALTHOUGH A DOCTOR'S LIFE was a busy one, there was always time to listen to my patients' various worries and woes, and I like to think that most of the people in my care left their consultation feeling greatly comforted and reassured. One frequent visitor to my surgery was a youth of some twenty years, who was unfortunately born with hydrocephalus – a condition in which there is an abnormal accumulation of fluid on the brain, commonly known as 'water on the brain'. He was a most likeable chap.

'People think that because I have such a large head, I must also have an enormous brain and that I ought to be Prime Minister or a genius,' he once told me. 'But I am really to be pitied, because I know most of it is water and that actually I have a very small brain. I can't think properly, nor can I earn my living.'

I felt downright sorry for this fellow, particularly as the only treatment available for his condition at the time was a largely ineffectual surgical procedure that carried with it a high mortality rate, but I enjoyed our talks and, however busy I was, I never turned him away.

At midday one winter's morning I was visiting an old lady who was recovering from an attack of pleurisy. She was a talkative soul and seemed to be very up-to-date with all the local gossip. We were sitting in the large lounge of one of the town's several boarding houses. Having completed our chat and my examination of her, I was about to leave when I noticed an old man with a long white beard sitting on his own at a table by a large bay window. He had a draughts board in front of him. Having occasionally played draughts, I wandered up to him and found that he was playing a game with himself.

'Isn't it rather difficult to play against yourself, when you know all the moves?' I asked him.

'Well,' he replied, 'I like the game and it passes the time away. I can't read much because I have cataracts in both eyes, but I can still see the pieces on the draughts board.'

Feeling sorry for the old man and, as it was only a quarter to one, I sat down and said, 'Come on, I will give you a game.'

'That's very kind of you,' he said.

We had not been playing for more than five minutes when he beat me decisively. 'I can't stand for that – let's have a return match,' I suggested.

In the meantime the boarding-house guests were congregating in the lounge before going into lunch. Several of them wandered over to the table where our game was in progress. Within a short time I was losing again. I remarked to one of the onlookers, a young woman, 'This old gentleman certainly plays a good game of draughts.'

'Do you know against whom you are playing?' she asked me.

'No,' I replied. 'I have only just made my friend's acquaintance.'

'Well,' she continued, 'he was once a draughts champion – isn't that correct, Grandpapa?'

'Yes,' he acknowledged modestly, 'I was a county champion for three successive years from 1903 to 1905.'

Considering I had been playing against a bona-fide draughts champion, I felt I had not played too badly.

*

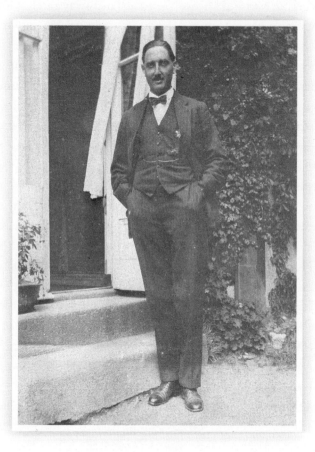

Outside my surgery, North Ford House, c.1920.

IT WAS DURING THE SUMMER that one of my most frustrating cases was finally solved: that of poor Betty Thompson. I was taking Nan and Michael on a short trip away and had hired a locum to cover for me. He arrived immaculately attired in a dark suit, beautifully ironed, striped trousers, patent-leather boots and spats. I thought he looked like the typical gigolo, but also thought he might go down well with my elderly spinsters. The morning we were leaving I showed him around the surgery and dispensary and briefed him on certain patients.

'You may well be called out tonight to a village where you will see a young girl who has vomited up a bowl of blood,' I warned him jokingly.

A few days into my holiday I received a letter from this locum, confirming that he had indeed got the call and that, as I had predicted, there was a large bowl of blood under the bed.

I also got a note from my surgery caretaker, Mr Densham, telling me that the locum had moved himself to one of the local hotels and had produced a wife! On my return I discovered that, instead of seeing to my patients' needs and doing patient visits in the afternoon, he and his wife took the river steamer for a pleasure trip, went shopping in a neighbouring town or went to a matinee performance at the local cinema.

The mystery of Betty was solved shortly after my return, when her mother was spotted coming back from the local abattoir with a bucket full of bullock's blood! Since her daughter's mysterious illness was well known locally, it was inevitable that people would put two and two together and that the gossip would soon reach me. After giving Mrs Thompson a good dressing-down, I suggested that she might like to change her doctor once more.

Many years later I heard that Betty was still in bed, but that the vomiting of blood had abruptly ceased. The strangest part about this case was the mutual conspiracy that existed between mother and daughter. I was puzzled both by Betty's complicity and by the sadistic pleasure that her mother seemed to take in keeping her daughter in bed. The mother clearly enjoyed the attention that we doctors continued to give her and her daughter; and, I suppose, the only way she could justify this was by faking the constant haemorrhages.

This was one mystery finally solved, but another, more intriguing one remains, which I cannot explain to this day. Dartmouth has a number of historic buildings dating back to the sixteenth and seventeenth centuries, and when I first arrived in the town there was a doctor living in one of these rather ancient-looking double-storeyed houses. As is the custom amongst medical men when establishing a practice in a new town, I paid regular courtesy calls on my medical colleagues, including this doctor.

What struck me as peculiar about his house was that the upper storey appeared much older than the ground floor, which was, of course, quite impossible. What gave it this appearance was that although the windows on the ground floor were made of modern plain-glass panes, the upper windows had diamond-shaped lead panes, such as were used hundreds of years earlier.

I called on this doctor late one afternoon at about 5.30 p.m. and was shown into his consulting room. We entered the room through a door from the hallway, and at the other end of the room was a green-baize door on a spring. I did not know at the time that this led into a small dispensary, with no other outlet apart from this one door.

Shortly before 6 p.m. I noticed the green-baize door opening slowly. Thinking this must be a patient coming to evening surgery, I jumped up, saying, 'I see your evening surgery has begun, so I will go.'

To my surprise my colleague shook his head and said, 'Oh, don't worry, please sit down – that's only the family ghost!'

'What do you mean?' I asked. 'Surely some pressure would be required to open that door, as I can see it is on a spring.'

'Yes, I know – you would think so,' said the doctor, 'but I can't explain it . . . Strange things do happen in this house. For instance, you wouldn't believe it, but sometimes we hear furniture being moved around in our lounge overhead, although when we go upstairs and look into the room, nothing appears to have moved from its usual position. Then, at other times, we hear footsteps on the staircase, although there is never anyone there. Anyway, as I have said, we have become quite used to these strange incidents.'

This doctor and his family left the town about a year or so later – perhaps they had had enough of these uncanny happenings – and a new doctor bought the practice. I met him in town a little while later, when he told me that his wife was due to be confined shortly and that the trained nurse they had booked to care for her had unfortunately been taken ill. Did I know of a reliable local midwife?

'Yes,' I said, 'she is very reliable and scrupulously clean. She must be about seventy years old and has been practising in this town for about half a century, during which time she has managed hundreds of confinements – many of them on her own. She uses Lysol antiseptic, wears rubber gloves and a long white coat, and though she is not hospital-trained, I would say she has more practical experience in bringing babies into the world than many a trained nurse.'

I gave the doctor the midwife's address and he duly booked her to attend to his wife. Some weeks later, when I arrived at my morning surgery, who should I see waiting for me but my old friend, the midwife. However, instead of the placid old dear whom I knew so well – for she had often assisted me – she looked quite pale and was trembling all over.

I said, 'Nurse, whatever is the matter with you?'

'Oh, Doctor,' she said, 'I left that doctor's house early this morning.'

'But his child was only born yesterday afternoon, so why ever did you leave so soon?'

'Oh, but that's a terrible, horrible house – I have never been so frightened in all my life. I could never go back there,' she exclaimed.

'My dear, do come and sit down and tell me what has happened,' I replied, astonished. This was her story.

'Well, the confinement was normal in all respects, and the doctor who was in attendance was perfectly satisfied with my work. In the evening we had tea and a little chat. Then, at about 9.30 p.m., the doctor suggested that we all have an early night.

They had made a bed for me in the little dressing room that opened onto his own and his wife's bedroom.

"'I will sleep in the large bedroom with my wife and baby," he said, "and should I want you during the night, I will call you."

'So after ensuring that mother and child were comfortable, I went into the dressing room and unpacked my clothes and placed them in a chest of drawers. Then, as was my usual custom, I read a magazine before putting out the light. The time must have been about 10 p.m. and I soon dropped off.

'I must have only been asleep for a couple of hours when I suddenly awoke and experienced the most horrible sensation of evil in the room. It was such a frightening feeling that I felt I must get up and go into my patient's bedroom and ask if I could possibly sleep in another room. Before I could move, suddenly all the bedclothes were pulled off the bed. I screamed out loud, and within seconds the doctor, who was a quick-tempered man, dashed into my room. He switched on the light, all the time cursing me for waking up his wife and baby and demanding to know what I meant by it! When I told him what had happened he said, "Nurse, you have had a bad nightmare; come into the bedroom and we will all have a cup of tea, and everything will be all right."

'He then got a torch, opened all the cupboards, including the wardrobe, looked under the bed and said: "Now, come along, Nurse, you can see there is no one in the room."

'I began to believe I must have dreamed it after all.

"'Now, to make things even safer," said the doctor, "I will lock our bedroom door, so no one can possibly get into your room without coming through our bedroom, and that will be impossible with the door locked. And what is more, I will give you the key of the dressing room, so you can lock yourself inside. Are you now satisfied?"

"'Yes, absolutely," I said.

'So after we had finished our tea, and feeling rather ashamed of myself, I went back to bed and fell asleep, having first locked the door from the inside.

'I don't know how long I had been asleep, but I was soon to wake again with that same dreadful feeling of evil in the room. Now I was panic-stricken, and my only thought was that I must somehow get into that other room, no matter what happened. I decided I would slowly slide myself to the side of the bed, unlock the door and rush into the big bedroom. However, no sooner had I reached the side of the bed than I felt two strong hands push me backwards. I yelled and yelled.

'The doctor came and banged on the door: "Open up, open up!" he shouted. "Switch on your bedside light!"

'I nearly passed out with fear, but managed to reach the light and switched it on. The hands had left my chest, and I could see there was no one in the room. After a while I was able to get out of bed and open the door. The doctor was in a violent temper and his first words were: "Nurse, you are fired!"

"'Don't worry," I said, "I am giving you notice. I am leaving at the first sign of daylight."

'So here I am,' the midwife said to me in a shaky voice. 'You know, Doctor, that house is haunted, if ever there was such a thing, and I don't know how any soul can live there.'

Well, it was not long before this story spread around the town, and apparently things got so bad in the house that shortly afterwards the doctor and his family left town. He could not sell his practice, as the house by then had such a fearsome reputation, and I heard that the Territorial Army eventually took it over as their local headquarters.

Years later I heard it was discovered that a murder had taken place in the dressing room some years previously. However, I could not imagine why a ghost – presumably the victim of the murder – should vent its wrath on a poor, harmless old midwife. Perhaps one of her ancestors had a hand in that murder: who knows?

As well as our home-grown ghosts, I also recall the macabre obsession of one of my patients – a very wealthy retired chocolate manufacturer – who lived in a village near us. He loved his garden, and his particular hobby was growing irises. He had a beautiful sunken garden with a pond and fountain in the middle of it. Around this there were irises of every colour and shape. He would point one out excitedly and say, 'This one is extremely valuable – worth twenty pounds!' Or 'This is a new hybrid from Japan, but I am not sure of its exact value.' Anyway, he had a very rare skin disease of his legs, and was delighted when I photographed them and wrote a description of them in a medical journal.

He had travelled a great deal. In his drawing room there was a glass showcase containing a variety of rare knick-knacks, but his gem, he said, was the mummified foot of an Egyptian child, which he had found on one of his wanderings near the

Pyramids. I admired it accordingly, though in truth I felt quite unnerved by it.

On one of my visits he told me that his wife had just the night before had a vivid dream of a native woman – possibly the mother of the footless child – standing at the end of her bed, pleading for the return of the foot. At this time there were sensational stories in the newspapers about the Curse of Tutankhamun, so perhaps unsurprisingly after her dream his wife desperately wanted him to return the little foot to Cairo Museum. Unfortunately for her peace of mind, my patient prized that little foot almost as much as his irises, so it never left the showcase.

At about the same time I used to attend an old naval pensioner and his wife. Situated in the middle of their mantelpiece was a beautiful Buddha, hand-painted in gold, crimson and blue. It was made of wood and appeared to be very old. I always admired it. On Christmas morning the old wife was taken ill with bronchitis, and so I was called out to their house. After attending to her, and as I was about to leave, she said, 'Doctor, we have a Christmas present for you!'

'How very kind,' I said, touched.

'Well, we want you to have that Buddha – the one you have always admired.'

'No,' I replied, 'that is far too generous of you, and I really could not accept that kind of gift, but if you do not want it, I would like to buy it from you.'

'Oh no!' she said. 'Look, here it is, all wrapped up and ready for you to take home. You have been most attentive and we would rather you have it, more than anyone else.'

She would not listen to my protests, so I took the Buddha home with me, thinking that it would be a nice surprise for Nan. Unfortunately she was horrified.

'Don't you know these Buddhas are terribly unlucky?' she asked. 'I couldn't possibly sleep with it in the house. Go and put it on the lawn, and then take it back to the old couple when you next visit them.'

A few days later I called round to see my patient again. By then she had completely recovered and answered my knock at the front door herself. When she saw me holding the Buddha, she screamed, 'Oh! Take it away, Doctor, take the horrible thing away!'

'But why?' I asked.

'Well, you see, ever since we have had it in this house, we have had the most terrible luck. We think there must be a curse on it.'

'Well, well,' I said, 'and you wanted to hand the bad luck on to your doctor!'

'But you've always admired it, Doctor. And when my husband came home before Christmas, I suggested we give it to you, thinking that you would be pleased and that our luck would turn. And, well, that's how it was.'

'However did you come to own it?' I asked her.

'When my husband was a young sailor, he was stationed on board a frigate up the Yangtze River. One day he saw the Buddha, slowly floating alongside his vessel, so he dived in and brought it back as a curio, but I curse the day it ever came into our house. It must have been stolen from a sacred temple,' she told me.

Now, where we lived in the town was very close to the River Dart, which is a tidal river, and I told my distressed patient that I had an idea.

'I happen to know the tide goes out at 8 p.m. this evening, so what we will do is jump into your husband's dinghy, row into the middle of the river and deposit the Buddha in the water.'

'Oh yes, Doctor, that is an excellent idea,' she said, looking relieved.

I called for her later that evening and, with both of us wrapped up against the cold night air, we duly set out in the dinghy. I rowed us out into the river and we gently set the Buddha down. There was just enough light from the town to let us see the figure start to drift slowly out to sea.

'Who knows?' I said. 'He will probably end up back in China in some fifty years' time. Anyway, I am quite sure you will have no further ill fortune now and will end your days quite happily.'

I numbered quite a few naval pensioners and their families among my patients because the Britannia Royal Naval College – the Royal Navy's prestigious training headquarters – was located in Dartmouth. The imposing red-brick buildings and clock tower sit high above the town and were built by the eminent architect, Sir Aston Webb, in the early 1900s. Prior to this, I believe all training took place on two old wooden sailing ships moored on the River Dart. One of them was the HMS *Britannia*, from which the college's name originates.

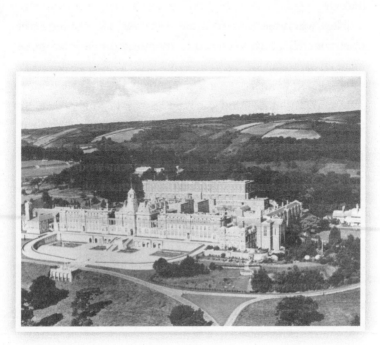

Dartmouth Naval College.

On one occasion I visited an old bachelor who was suffering from gout. What intrigued me was not his medical condition, which was really quite common, but his amazing array of antique china and Staffordshire pottery. He seemed to be quite an authority and proudly showed me his collection while explaining how each of the pieces came to be in his possession.

On asking him what he considered his best piece and the one he prized most, he remarked, 'Oh, that's easy, it's down in that cupboard over there – do take it out and have a look at it.'

When I opened the cupboard he was pointing at, I saw at once by the china handle that the piece in question was a chamber pot.

I turned to him and said, 'Are you pulling my leg?'

'Not at all. Please take it out and have a good look at it.'

When I removed the chamber pot, I was amazed to see that the rim and bottom were surrounded by a twist of golden oak leaves and that on one side of the chamber was the royal coat of arms. On the other side were three white feathers with the words *Ich Dien* – meaning 'I serve' – printed beneath them.

'What exactly is this?' I asked.

'Do you realize, Doctor, that you are holding the very chamber pot used every night by Edward VII, King of England?' asked my patient, smiling. 'I was his personal orderly on the *Britannia* when he was Prince of Wales and, after he left the ship, I took the jerry [chamber pot]. I wouldn't sell it for a thousand guineas, though I suppose it ought to be in the British Museum!'

'Our family held your grandfather in very high esteem. My mother often mentioned him as my grandmother was a local midwife and she knew him very well.'

ERIC HANNAFORD, 2012

7

'Tell Me, Doctor, Are You Saved?'

The Unexpected in Birth and Death

'WELL, MRS WILLIAMS, let us see what the manometer reading is today,' I said. She bared her left arm and I put the rubber cuff around it and began blowing up the pressure to take a systolic and diastolic reading.

Mrs Williams was an elderly lady of some threescore years and ten, who had been under my care for about two years. She suffered from occasional attacks of giddiness and occipital neuralgia, and by now her memory was starting to fail. She was also suffering from arteriosclerosis – thickening and hardening of the walls of the cerebral blood vessels – which is very common in old age. For a few months now she had had very high blood pressure and, as was her wont, she came in to see me about every three months to have it measured. On this occasion she was in my consulting room happily chatting away, and apparently in very good health.

'Oh, Doctor, my left arm has gone to sleep,' she said suddenly, and a few seconds later, 'and now my fingers are tingling!'

I quickly removed the cuff from her arm, but as I did so she fell off the chair and onto the floor. With the aid of my receptionist we quickly lifted her onto the couch. I immediately sent for the ambulance to take her to hospital, but she died before transport arrived. Unfortunately I had witnessed a massive cerebral haemorrhage, for which no treatment could be applied.

Her sudden death was a shock, but I have never forgotten another, much stranger case that I once had. In our town there were two undertakers, whose respective firms appeared to flourish. At Christmas time bottles of whisky were sent as gifts to us doctors, with their compliments – I presume for all the business we had given them during the year.

At 6.25 a.m. one day I received an urgent phone call to tell me that one of the town's undertakers – a patient of mine – had suffered a heart attack, and would I come round immediately? I arrived to find the man lying on his lounge floor. I tried artificial respiration, injections of heart stimulants and cardiac massage, but there was no sign of life. It was too late to save him. I therefore sent, at the request of his distraught wife, for the town's second undertaker, a short, rather stout little man, whom I did not know at all.

When he arrived and saw that it was his rival lying on the

ground – for there was always great competition between them – his eyes twinkled and I could see that he now felt he truly had charge of all the local townspeople's last journey to the grave.

'Well,' he said insincerely, as he studied his dead adversary, 'this is a bad business' – though to him, of course, it meant good business!

'Yes,' I agreed, 'I have seen quite a few of these coronary-thrombosis cases over the last few years. Let us move him from the floor and place him on his bed.'

So, with some difficulty and heavy breathing on the part of the second undertaker, we lifted my dead patient by his legs and shoulders and carried him to his bedroom. I did not know at the time that Undertaker No. 2 also suffered from a weak heart. However, having measured up my patient and finished with the other formalities, he went downstairs to console the wife and make arrangements for the funeral. While he was away I wrote out my late patient's death certificate.

Coming back upstairs, Undertaker No. 2 and I had a little chat and then he looked at his watch and, seeing that he was late for some appointment, quickly stooped down to pick up a rather heavy-looking bag. As he straightened up he dropped the bag, clasped his hands to his chest, gave a loud groan and fell down dead at my feet.

I must say, the shock unnerved me for a moment, but then I got busy trying to revive this sudden new patient of mine. All to no avail. Here I was, with two dead undertakers, who had died within an hour of each other in the same room and possibly even from the same complaint. Surely a unique happening!

With some difficulty, after he had heard my story, I managed to obtain the services of another undertaker from a neighbouring town. Meanwhile, I called Undertaker No. 2's wife to tell her of the tragedy. She came straight over and, after doing my best to console both these recent widows, I left them weeping on each other's shoulders.

Sadly, a doctor knows only too well that it is often impossible to save a life. When I first began to study medicine in 1910, no specific treatment had been discovered for many of the infectious diseases that plagued mankind. It is true there were serums available for the treatment of diphtheria, tetanus and other fevers, but they were mostly ineffectual. In my early days as a GP in Devon I remember using the anti-pneumococcal serum in the treatment of pneumonia, and anti-streptococcal serum for septicaemia, but their curative powers seemed negligible. The cocci diseases, such as boils, pneumonia, septicaemia, gonorrhoea and scarlet fever, and bacillary diseases such as tuberculosis and typhoid were frequently fatal.

I had a patient, a lovely girl called Rose, who was twenty years old and who had been a panel patient of mine for a few years. She had no memories of her mother as the poor woman had died of consumption, which is what we called tuberculosis when it affected the lungs. There was no cure for TB in those days. Rose was just three years old when her mother died and, as a result, her aunt, who ran a small village post office outside Dartmouth, had brought her up as her own child. Unfortunately when Rose was ten she developed tuberculosis of her right hip, and so this leg was three inches shorter than the left one and she wore a boot with a three-inch sole to make up the difference. Not only was Rose the most popular girl in the village, but she was also very pretty and had the sweetest nature. She was, quite simply, adored by all those who knew her.

One Sunday morning she started to feel unwell and complained of severe abdominal pain. Her aunt said she would phone for the doctor, but Rose refused, telling her aunt that she did not wish to trouble the doctor on a Sunday. So she went to bed and put a hot-water bottle on her side. As she seemed much worse in the morning, her aunt insisted on calling me and I went at once. I could see that Rose was gravely ill: her abdomen was as hard as a board, and I diagnosed a burst appendix and peritonitis. I did not wish to waste time waiting for an ambulance, so I took her and her aunt with me in my car to the hospital, where we operated on her within an hour. Her abdomen was full of pus, and all we could do was put in drainage pipes.

Rose made a remarkable recovery, but later her TB hip flared up again and she had a recurrence of peritonitis – this time, I presume, of a tubercular nature. Unfortunately these were the days before sulphonamides and antibiotics and, in spite of every care and all possible treatment, Rose's condition deteriorated day by day. On the Sunday morning, as I examined her, I felt sure she was going to die before midnight. I telephoned her aunt and asked that she come to the hospital as soon as possible. The toxins of the peritonitis had paralysed all of her abdominal nerves, and I told the aunt that Rose was free of pain and suffering, but that her heart was giving out. The aunt came and spent the day with her.

I visited Rose for the third time that day, just after tea, when she was asking her aunt to take a length of material from her chest of drawers at home, which she wanted made into a skirt, as she thought she would be well enough to attend the village dance the following month. When her aunt heard this, she looked at me as if I was out of my mind – telling her that Rose only had a few hours to live, and yet here was the dear girl, planning what she was going to wear to the Christmas dance!

Rose was sitting up with a bed-rest and several pillows behind her. She was in the general ward and we had put screens around her. Sitting beside her bed were her aunt, the hospital matron, the ward sister and me. All of a sudden she stopped talking to us – a beatific smile came over her face, she held her arms out as if about to embrace someone and said, 'Mummy, I am just coming!'

She then fell back dead on the pillows, a smile still radiating her face. I am afraid we were all in tears. I am sure that at the moment of death Rose had a vision of her mother, whom she never knew, calling for her.

IN MAY 1926 Nan told me that she was expecting again, and we looked forward to another addition to our family. Michael was very excited to hear that he would have a brother or sister to play with. He was five years old at the time, and in a year or so would begin his formal education at Park House Preparatory School in Paignton.

News of another pregnancy – a rather less expected one than our own – sticks in my mind from around this time. I was examining the dislocated cartilage on a patient's knee one morning when there was a loud banging on my consulting-room door. I heard a woman shouting at my receptionist that she must see the doctor at once. Thinking someone had committed suicide – or murder – and that the case was most urgent, I asked my patient with the knee trouble to return temporarily to the waiting room while I found out what all the fuss was about.

No sooner had I opened the door than a strange woman burst into the room and flung herself onto my examination couch.

'Doctor,' she pleaded, 'tell me, please, does the "change of life" give you kicks in the stomach?'

'Not as a rule,' I said, 'but let me examine you.'

'I am nearly fifty,' she said. 'I have had no periods for five months, and all my friends say, "What do you expect, dearie – you have the change of life, dearie." But in the last few days I have had the most peculiar sensations in my tummy.'

'Please lie down,' I told her. I could see her shaking as I examined her, already knowing what I was most likely to find. 'Yes, I would say you are nearly five months pregnant.'

'Oh, Doctor, no, that can't be right,' she protested. 'I can't possibly have a baby now. You see, I have two grown-up children – a son of twenty-eight and a daughter of twenty-six.'

Well, I told my new patient to try and stay calm as there was nothing that could be done about it, and she would just have to accept her situation.

'I don't know what my husband will say,' she told me as she left, still looking rather dazed.

'I am sure he will be very happy,' I replied, hoping I was correct.

Her pregnancy was trouble-free and, some months later, she had a normal confinement. The baby daughter I delivered was her most precious jewel, doted on by all the family.

EARLY ONE MORNING I received a frantic message from a patient to say that he could not wake his wife, and lying on the floor beside the bed was an empty bottle that had contained sleeping pills.

'Please can you come at once, Doctor,' he begged.

My patient and his wife had recently come to England from the Far East and seemed to be a very wealthy couple. I had visited them once before, and we had chatted about their travels and they had shown me the large amount of oriental furniture and antiques which they had collected along the way; amongst them was a set of William and Mary chairs, a Queen Anne settee, a beautiful grandfather clock and a huge burnished gong.

When I entered the patient's bedroom I found her in a coma and breathing loudly. I shook her and I pinched her arms, but she remained deeply unconscious. I gave her an enema of black coffee. I passed a stomach pump. I injected her with stimulants and, after about half an hour, there were some slight signs of returning consciousness.

'Bring that gong up from the hall,' I said to my patient's husband, 'and please ask your butler to come up to the bedroom. Now,' I explained, 'I am going to get your wife out of bed, and you and I will walk her up and down the bedroom, and each time we reach the end of the room I want your butler to strike that gong as hard as he can.'

Within five minutes, as the gong boomed out, my patient gave a jump – she could obviously hear the sound. We continued to walk her up and down for what seemed like hours. Every now and then the butler would relieve one of us and the odd man out would be the gong-beater. By lunchtime the patient was almost conscious, and when I finally left the house at teatime she was normal in all respects. She told me that taking too many pills had been an accident and vowed to be more careful in the future.

This story continued till Christmas morning, when we had just had breakfast at home and I was upstairs, playing with Michael. There was a ring at the front door and our maid looked out of the window and saw a man with a hand-barrow outside, on which was a long and narrow oblong box covered by a sheet.

Rushing upstairs to find me, she said breathlessly, 'Oh, Doctor, there's a man brought a coffin for you. He's waiting outside.'

In the meantime our neighbours across the street were looking out of their window and saying to one another, 'How terribly sad. Who could have died in the doctor's house, and on Christmas Day of all days?'

I opened the window and shouted to the man with the barrow, 'I'm very sorry, but we don't want any coffins here on Christmas Day, thank you.'

'Oh, but it *is* for you, Doctor, and I have a letter here that is addressed to you.'

'Nonsense,' I said, 'there must be some mistake.'

Anyway, I thought I had better go downstairs and deal with it. I opened the letter, which read:

Dear Doctor,

I can never forget how you saved my wife's life, and we can never forget the debt of gratitude we owe you, and hope you will accept this grandfather clock as a Christmas gift.

Unlike the gift of the Buddha some years earlier, Nan allowed me to keep the clock!

About six weeks after this, on 11 February 1927, our daughter Althea Rosemary was born. When Nan went into labour, we sent for our doctor and waited . . . and waited. We were experiencing a bitterly cold spell and he had been delayed by the weather. In the end I had to step in and attend to the birth myself.

Fortunately for Nan, Althea was a much smaller baby than her brother Michael had been and there were no complications, but I do recall that Nan was not at all amused when I began to

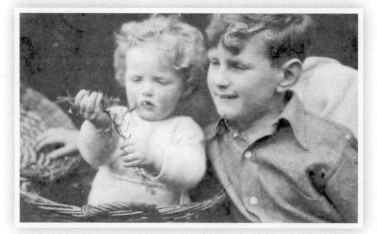

Little Althea with Michael, 1928.

giggle uncontrollably about halfway through the proceedings. However, all's well that ends well!

'TELL ME, DOCTOR, are you saved?'

I had just had a tooth filled by my dentist and was about to leave his surgery when he asked me this. As I hesitated, not knowing what he meant and unsure how to respond, he added, 'Saved in Christ I mean.'

'How kind of you to take such an interest in my religious welfare,' I replied cautiously.

'Not at all, Doctor,' he said, handing me a wad of papers. 'Do take these tracts away with you, study them well, and I am confident you will be saved.'

It so happened that one of my lady patients, who subsequently visited the dentist some time later, did not get off as lightly as I did.

'Mrs Matthews,' said the dentist, as he completed a filling, 'are you saved in Christ?'

'Yes, I think so,' said my patient.

'No, Mrs Matthews, you don't think about it – you are either saved or not saved. Now, please take these tracts with you, study them well and by the time you come in for your next appointment on Friday morning, I know you will be saved.'

'It was very kind of you to let me read those religious articles,' said my patient when she entered the dentist's room the following Friday. 'I really think I am saved.'

'Oh dear, oh dear – *think, think,*' said the dentist. 'I told you, you don't think about this, you are either saved or you are not. You know it; you don't *think* about it! Now at 5 p.m. this afternoon we have a prayer meeting in our church hall – I will take you down there in my car; my friends will all pray for your salvation, and you will know Christ and your sins will be forgiven.'

Mrs Matthews, being a kind and gentle lady and not wishing to disappoint the dentist, agreed to attend the prayer meeting. As the members of the congregation left, the dentist joyfully came up to her, telling her that he knew she was saved.

'This time,' said my patient, 'I really think I am saved.'

'No, Mrs Matthews! I have told you before: you do not think about so serious a matter – there is only one thing left for you to do. I ask you to go down on your knees for an hour in this church and pray for your delivery from this sinful world. I have to go back to my surgery for half an hour for an appointment, but I will lock you in the hall so that no one can disturb you, and I will return and take you home in my car within the hour.'

Now, by an extraordinary coincidence, who should the dentist meet as he was walking back to his surgery but Mrs Matthews' husband, who had been out of town on business for the whole day. Addressing the husband, he said, 'Major Matthews, I am extremely happy to tell you your wife has been saved!'

'Good gracious, has she been in an accident?' the husband asked, instantly alarmed.

'No, no, she is alive and well, but she is saved in Christ. She is quite safe, locked up in our church in prayer.'

I don't know exactly what the husband said to the dentist, but he told me later he was furious and almost knocked him down there and then. 'Take me down to your church hall and set my wife free immediately!' he demanded.

After that unfortunate set of circumstances the dentist's practice deteriorated rapidly, as all and sundry were accosted in the streets and asked if they were saved in Christ. It was a terribly sad case, and eventually our dentist had to be sent to an asylum as a case of religious mania.

Just as sad was the case of one of our local businessmen. He was a most respected member of the community and active in town affairs. Although he had never been elected to the high office of mayor, many thought he would have been ideal, as he was always pleasant, courteous and tactful with everybody. I knew him as both a patient and as a friend.

Suddenly he was struck down with misfortune.

I was holding my morning surgery and was in the middle of examining a patient when my friend suddenly burst into my consulting room. Before I could react, he grasped my two hands and said excitedly, 'Doc, you can get rid of all your old patients. From now on you will be my private physician, at ten thousand pounds a year. I am going to buy you a Rolls-Royce motor car and I am going to build a new house for you, as the one you live in is quite unsuitable for my private physician.'

'But . . . ' was as far as I got, before he was off again.

'No, no, Doc, it is the only thing to do. Quite frankly, I am so wealthy I could buy up the whole town, but I do not wish to do this at present. I have, however, bought up all the almshouses in Dartmouth so that there will be no more poor people in the town, and I have purchased all the motor boats in the harbour. I have also organized a formal lunchtime banquet for the Mayor and council at the Majestic Hotel tomorrow at 12.30 p.m., and of course you, Doc, as my private physician, will be my honoured guest.'

While he continued to rant, the patient I had been attending to slipped out of my consulting room – and quite what he told the patients in the waiting room I can't begin to imagine. I immediately came to the conclusion that my friend was raving mad, but I had no difficulty getting rid of him as he told me he had to telephone all the town councillors to invite them to his luncheon party. In the meantime I tried to telephone his wife at their home, but there was no reply.

I continued seeing all my other patients throughout the morning, when suddenly the wife turned up, and what a sorry tale she had to tell me! Apparently he had behaved most peculiarly all morning and after lunch had gone to his bank where, by cheque, he had withdrawn about a hundred pounds' worth of sixpences and threepenny pieces. He had then wandered through the streets scattering the coins about the pavements. The local school had just ended for the day, and soon hoards of children were running alongside him picking up the coins as they were thrown about. It reminded me of the story of the Pied Piper of Hamelin.

Anyway, eventually he returned home and his wife telephoned me to let me know. I immediately went up to their house along with two medical colleagues. After examining our friend, we all came to the conclusion that in his youth he must have contracted syphilis, although during the many years that he had prospered in business, no symptoms had been manifest. General paralysis of the insane – or GPI, as it is commonly known among the medical fraternity – is a later complication of the disease. Patients afflicted with it frequently develop symptoms later on in life; they have the most grandiose ideas and everything appears exaggerated. For instance, if one was to ask one of these unfortunates with whom he lunched and what was on the menu, he is as likely as not to say: 'Oh! I lunched with God, and we had elephant chops!' The delusion that our old friend produced was that he had suddenly acquired great wealth – he was, as far as he was concerned, a millionaire.

There was no cure and we knew his condition would only worsen, inevitably leading to dementia and death. It was a terribly sad case. We had to sign him up as insane and he was taken to the asylum that same evening.

'We lived at 4 Charles Street. Dr White-Cooper brought me into the world in September 1931 and he was my doctor until the day he left Dartmouth in 1949. He was a very kind man, a real charmer, and as a young girl I used to think he was so handsome. Before I was born, he used to visit my granny Annie Perring every day, as she had what they called in those days "water on the brain". Apparently, he was very good to her and would recommend that she drank a sherry-glass of milk stout each day, and he would even put a poker in it, to warm it up for her. She died in 1930 aged fifty-four. He also looked after me when I had the mumps.'

MYRA GALLOWAY, 2012

8

'Drinking Bovril Will Not Cure Lumbago'

The Power of the Mind

'Is this the doctor, then?' old Albert asked. 'Would you believe me, Doctor, if I said I haven't had to see a medical man for ninety years! Not since I was a lad. And now I'm a hundred.'

'That is indeed remarkable,' I agreed. 'There are many who would like to know your secret – myself included!'

I had been asked to examine Albert, who lived on a farm some eight miles from my surgery. He had luxurious white side-whiskers, but his upper lip and chin were shaved, and in general he was very spry and alert. He lay on his bed as I examined him and pointed to a letter hanging on the wall above him, in a gilt frame.

'Do you see that letter, Doctor?' he said proudly. 'There's not many can say King George has written to them.'

I looked and saw the signature 'George R. I.' Apparently King

George V had been a cadet at the Royal Naval College and had frequently had tea with old Albert on his farm. Now Albert, at his great age, was still riding to hounds. He had an old white mare, onto which he was hoisted by two of his farm labourers. He was unable to sit up straight, but would lie forward over the mare's neck. After the meet the old mare would always find her way home, and my patient's farm labourers would be there to lift him off his steed. When King George V heard that he had ridden to hounds on his one-hundredth birthday, he sent Albert a personal letter, which, as I had seen, was greatly prized.

Albert had a small hernia, which had apparently been troubling him for many years. At his age an operation would have been inadvisable, so I explained to him that a truss would keep his rupture in place. I also asked him if I could examine his heart. My stethoscope greatly intrigued him and, as I sounded his chest and heard his old heart beating lub-dup, lub-dup, perfectly regularly, I thought to myself how extraordinary and amazing to hear those two sounds due to the heart's contractions, which has been beating like this for more than one hundred years without rest. No man-made machine, I thought, had been invented that would work so perfectly and so long without attention.

I asked Albert what he ate, wondering if that might hold the key to his longevity. His main diet appeared to be eggs, meat, cheese and cider.

Having measured him for his special hernia support, I brought it out some ten days later and showed him how to put it on. Sadly I didn't see him again, and old Albert never lived to see his 101st birthday. He died of a seizure a few months later.

IN THE EARLY 1930S, during the Depression years, some of my patients found it hard to make ends meet. In fact this was the case even before the Depression, but it did seem that life became much noticeably harder for many then. When some of my patients were unable to pay my medical fees, they would instead give me gifts of eggs, ducks, pheasants, milk or potatoes. However, this was not the case with one particular family – they were a queer lot, quite unsophisticated, but extremely wealthy.

Mrs Hill was a widow of ninety-three. In spite of her age she was active, well organized and very shrewd. She ruled the roost. She owned one of the largest and most prosperous farms in the district, and had two sons – Billy and George. She also had a daughter, who was slightly unhinged and seemed to be the family drudge. They were all completely illiterate. Mother took charge of the purse strings. The family trusted neither the stock exchange nor the banks. In fact I doubt if they had ever heard of the former, so their earnings were never invested. Accordingly Mrs Hill only believed in solid gold, and this was stored in small bags in a huge safe. One day, while I was visiting the farm, she was counting her money with the safe door open and there, like an Aladdin's cave, were rows upon rows of little bags, all filled with gold sovereigns.

Billy and George, both in their early sixties, were successful farmers who had won many prizes at the county agricultural shows. They spoke with a typical Devonshire jargon – never using the pronoun 'I'; it was always 'us'. George looked like a real John Bull with his Norfolk jacket, riding breeches and gaiters. He was very popular, whereas Billy was shy and reserved. On several occasions I went to partridge shoots in their stubble fields, and George was a first-class shot. Billy was a great patron of the local beagles, and hunting the elusive hare was his only pastime.

The interior of the farmhouse was a shambles. Pigs and poultry wandered in and out of the kitchen. The rooms were unkempt; sacks littered the floor, instead of carpets. On the walls were a few hunting scenes.

Now to their mother, her three offspring – as this story will show – were still young children. One day I was called to see George, who was in bed, lying on his stomach; he had a large abscess on his buttock – a painful condition – that required opening and draining, but it presented no real danger. On leaving, I went into the kitchen, which they generally used as a dining room, to tell Mother about George, and there I found the old lady weeping copiously.

'What's wrong, my dear?' I asked, taken aback.

'It's my boy, my George,' she sobbed. 'Us know us'll never rear him!'

George was now more than sixty years old – how perfectly sweet!

On another occasion the elder brother, Billy, was laid low with a severe attack of lumbago. Mother treated him with herbal remedies, but to no avail. The pain increased and Billy took to his bed.

'You must have Doctor, see,' George told him. 'I shall go to the post office and telephone Dr White-Cooper.'

Unlike his brother George, Billy was morose, crafty and suspicious – a crabbed old bachelor. He did not have a high regard for the medical profession and frequently told me so – in so many words! All his teeth had been removed at some time, except for one central lower incisor. This used to waggle about, and many times I would say: 'Come on, Billy, let's get this last one out!'

But no, he refused to part with it. How he managed to chew his food was always a mystery to me.

'Hello, Billy,' I said, 'what's wrong with you? This is the first time I've ever seen you in bed.'

'Yes,' he said, 'I've a bad pain here, see.' He pointed to the lower part of his back as he turned over onto his side.

'It's nothing to be concerned about, Billy – it's probably only an attack of lumbago, and I will soon have you up and about again in a few days.'

'Us'll see, us'll see,' muttered the disbelieving Billy.

I administered some analgesia and told him to remain in bed and that I would visit him again in a day or two.

On my next visit he didn't seem to be in too good a mood.

'Well, how are you, Billy?'

'Us no better, us no better. Us don't think much of your stuff, us don't think.'

'I've had a brainwave,' I said. 'I'll send you out a new treatment and, when I see you next, I am sure you will be up and walking about again.'

'Us'll see, us'll see,' said the unconvinced Billy.

When I visited him again a few days later I was pleased to see him stumping round the house with his old stick.

'There you are, Billy, I told you this new treatment would soon cure you.'

'T'aint your stuff,' said Billy, pointing to the mantelpiece. 'Parson sent it, see – wonderful stuff, wonderful stuff.'

On the mantelpiece stood a half-empty jar of Bovril.

'Billy,' I said, 'drinking Bovril will not cure lumbago.'

'Drinking it, be damned,' he said, 'it's liniment, and Mother has rubbed my back with it. Wonderful stuff, wonderful stuff – that parson's far cleverer than you doctors!'

As you may imagine, Billy's shirt and the bed sheets were in a terrible mess.

'Never mind, Mother will soon put that to rights,' said Billy.

Being unable to read, the old mother had clearly thought that the vicar had sent up a bottle of liniment, which she had rubbed vigorously into Billy's painful back, with the most remarkable curative effect. It was another instance of a faith-cure, and of mind over matter.

The power of mind over matter – and of hypnotism – has fascinated me ever since I was a young boy. We know that if someone is put into a hypnotic state, they do not appear to feel pain, and as a child in South Africa I once observed the most amazing case of this nature. I saw a wizened old Malay, seated trance-like in a chair, open his mouth and allow a fellow countryman to drop a small red-hot coal into his mouth. No sooner had the coal entered his mouth than steam issued from it, whereupon the old man removed the piece of black coal, apparently feeling none the worse for wear. His throat and mouth were examined by torchlight and revealed no swelling or redness anywhere. This must surely represent terrific concentration of mind over matter.

Even harder to explain is the story of a well-known Egyptian fakir who was buried alive in a coffin for twenty-eight days and then disinterred, whereupon he sat up, apparently none the worse for his lengthy sleep. At the time sceptics claimed he must have had an oxygen tube let down underground, but to prove this false he then had a glass coffin made, in which he lay for twenty-eight days at the bottom of a swimming pool, where he could be seen by all and sundry. From a medical point of view I do not understand how any human being can exist for so long without oxygen. The medical profession is taught that the brain requires a good supply of oxygen in order to function, and that changes to the supply of oxygen (or a reduction of it) can have serious, if not fatal, consequences. The fakir's heart must beat, otherwise his blood would clot, but the deficiency in oxygen is what baffled the medical fraternity. This Egyptian fakir explained that he had swallowed his tongue, thus closing his larynx, and then put himself into a trance using autosuggestion.

Whatever the truth of that story, I have had many opportunities to witness hypnotists practising on others. In fact an American hypnotist arrived in Dartmouth and was to perform at our local club. He asked for a volunteer who would be willing to be put into a trance for one week. At the end of the week the volunteer would be taken onto the club's stage, where he would be awoken and presented by the town's mayor with a cheque for twenty pounds – which, considering this was quite some time ago, was a large sum of money.

There were apparently several volunteers and, once a suitable subject was found, he was duly put into a cataleptic trance – the deepest form of hypnosis. I remember that there was a roster, and club members were scheduled to watch the subject each hour of every day. The subject took neither food nor drink, nor passed any urine during the whole week. When he was carried onto the stage, he appeared to be as stiff as a steel rod. His head was placed on one chair, his heels on a second, and then the hypnotist stood on his subject; and finally, with a sledgehammer, he broke a small paving stone on the unfortunate man's abdomen. The volunteer was then brought out of his trance and quickly revived, seemingly none the worse for his recent ordeal. He was loudly cheered by the audience and presented with his cheque by our mayor.

Not everyone can be hypnotized. You cannot hypnotize an imbecile or a young child, for they will not listen to you or concentrate on what you are saying, so all suggestion made by the hypnotist is wasted. However, once someone has been hypnotized it is not difficult to put them into the hypnotic state again.

This is exactly what happened when I once attended a hypnotic show. On the stage there were six subjects, sitting on numbered chairs, and each one had been hypnotized. During the interval the hypnotist told them all to go back to their seats in the audience, but he also said that when the curtains opened, whether they liked it or not, all six of them would automatically return to their seats on the stage. Now it happened that Number Six was a university student, and he rejoined his two friends in the audience, who were sitting in seats next to mine.

'John, how much of the show have you seen?' they asked him.

He thought for a moment and said, 'I've been asleep, haven't I?'

'You fool,' they said, 'you have paid to see this show, and yet you are one of its stars and you have been amusing us with your antics. For goodness' sake, make up your mind to stay here and see the second half.'

'By Jove, I will,' he said.

The curtains opened and the other five subjects walked up to the stage and sat on their appropriate chairs.

'Come on, Number Six, hurry up,' said the hypnotist, 'we can't run the show without you.'

But Number Six stayed where he was, muttering to himself, 'I am not going up – nothing will make me go up. I am staying right here!'

His friends agreed that he should stay with them, but the hypnotist was having none of it and, not having verbally persuaded Number Six to return to the stage, walked slowly down the aisle towards John. When he was about a yard away he put up his hand and said, 'Sleep.' Number Six fell back, as if shot, and then duly got up and followed the hypnotist to his seat on the stage.

I found out at first hand that I too made an excellent subject for hypnotism, having travelled to London to see a very famous hypnotist from the continent who was giving a show at Earls Court. While standing in the queue waiting to buy tickets, I recognized a man standing in front of me as the hypnotist from another show that I had recently seen.

'Isn't this a busman's holiday for you?' I asked him.

He looked at me strangely and said, 'I don't know you, do I?'

'Not personally no, but I was in the audience of one of your shows a few months ago,' I replied.

'Well, this continental hypnotist is internationally renowned, and I'm hoping to pick up a few tips from him,' said the man in the queue. He looked at his watch and said, 'Come on, we have about twenty-five minutes before the show starts – let's go to the bar and have a drink.'

I went along with him, he hypnotized me and I paid for the drinks!

A PATIENT OF MINE, knowing of my great interest in hypnotism, once related this very strange story to me, which he assured me was true.

'Many years ago,' he said, 'I lived in London and was advised to see a doctor for an internal complaint. A friend of mine said, "The man you absolutely must see is quite outstanding." I looked up this doctor's name in the *Medical Directory* and he appeared to have every known medical degree. He was obviously a super-specialist. When I entered his consulting room, I saw his nurse sitting on a chair beside him.

'The super-specialist told me, "I am rather unorthodox in my methods. You see, I do not have to examine you to diagnose your case. I put my nurse, sitting beside me, into an hypnotic trance and then, in this condition, she diagnoses your case."

'"Fantastic," I said.

'"Yes, it is remarkable, isn't it?" said the super-specialist.

'The nurse then left the chair and lay on a couch behind a screen. I could hear the doctor suggesting to the nurse in a droning voice that she was getting more and more drowsy, and then he finally said, "Major Castle is sitting in my room. Tell me, Nurse, what do you consider his illness to be? On hearing his symptoms, please diagnose his case."

'The nurse then spoke very slowly and said, "Major Castle is suffering from a mild attack of cholecystitis, an inflammation of the gall bladder." Subsequently this was found to be clinically correct and, with the necessary treatment, I soon recovered.

'Some months later, one winter's morning, I was at the St James's Club, of which I was a member, and saw a small crowd huddled around the fireplace. Who should be in the midst but my old friend and super-specialist Dr Black Magic, as he came to be known. He was explaining to those around him the wonderful hypnotic power he had over his nurse.

'"Do you know," he said, "I can put my nurse into a trance and tell her to follow one of you fellows tonight, and she will tell me exactly where you are going and what you are doing."

'"That's impossible," argued one of the members. "In fact, I will bet you" – and he named a figure – "that your nurse will not be able to follow me tonight."

"'I will take on the bet," said Dr Black Magic, "and I'll tell you what I'll do. At 7 p.m. tonight I will put my nurse into a deep hypnotic trance, and tell her I want her to follow you and record exactly what you are doing at the time you are doing it. I should like two members of the club to come to my rooms as witnesses, and for them to take down particulars of your evening's activities, and I would like two other members of the club to accompany you, wherever you choose to go. Then I would like us to meet here again tomorrow evening at 6 p.m., when I will read out what my nurse has said. Then you can pay up your bet," said the doctor, with a chuckle.

'Well,' my patient continued, 'we all met at the pre-arranged time at the club the following evening, and Dr Black Magic read out exactly what the nurse dictated while in a trance, with the two club members acting as witnesses: "You and your two friends have hailed a taxi. You are now travelling up Regent Street. You have decided to go to Driver's for oysters. You are now dining on oysters and stout and brown bread" – pause – "You have hailed another taxi; you are now travelling up Shaftesbury Avenue to the Palace Theatre, where you are seeing a play" – named – "You are now sitting in seats sixteen, seventeen and eighteen in the second row of the Dress Circle" – pause – "At the interval you have gone to the bar; you are drinking whisky and soda; you are returning to your seats" – pause – "The show is over; you have hailed another taxi, you and your friends have driven to a" – named – "where a cabaret is in progress" – named – "On the menu you are having the following dishes; you are now having" – named; pause – "You are now having the second course" – named; pause – "You are now having coffee and a Benedictine liqueur. You have said goodbye to your friends and are going home by tube railway."'

The report was correct in every single detail and Dr Black Magic collected his bet, to the amazement of all the club members, and especially the victim of this uncanny incident. Fortunately Dr Black Magic handed over the bet money to the club's treasurers for one of its charities, so at least some good came of it.

Less controversially, I did find a way to help one of my patients using hypnotism. One market day afternoon a farmer's wife brought her seventeen-year-old daughter to see me, with the story that her daughter had been out milking the cows the evening before, but when she returned to the house, she told her mother that her right arm had suddenly become fixed and she was unable to straighten it. Her mother rubbed some liniment into it, but it was to no avail and she told her daughter to go to bed and that, when she awoke in the morning, it would probably be quite normal again. However, this was not the case and all through the night and the following morning the girl's arm remained tightly flexed.

I examined the girl and then asked if she would leave the room, as I wished to have a chat with her mother. As soon as she did so, I said to the mother, 'Do you know, I don't believe there is anything physically wrong with your daughter. I think she has what is known as a hysterical spasm.'

'What do you mean, Doctor? My daughter hysterical? Absolute nonsense! How can you say such a thing? I am going to go and see another doctor.'

'You are most welcome,' I said patiently. 'If it makes you feel any better, why not try two or three.'

With that, the mother picked up her bag and stamped out of the room.

A few hours later this lady returned. She immediately said, 'I have come to apologize to you, Doctor. The two doctors I have seen have said exactly the same thing as you. Please will you help us?'

'All right,' I agreed. 'I suggest you bring your daughter into hospital tomorrow. We will give her a general anaesthetic and I am sure the spasm will disappear.'

The girl was accordingly anaesthetized and, as I expected, the arm relaxed and became quite straight, but no sooner was she conscious again than it became tightly flexed once more. Now I was in a real quandary. Understandably the mother was deeply disappointed and asked me what else I could suggest.

'Hypnotism is the answer,' I replied.

Now it so happened that living next to us at the time was a retired clergyman, who had a reputation for successfully treating people using medical hypnosis. I took my young patient to see him the following day and while she was in a deep trance, and using strong post-hypnotic suggestion that the arm would never again become rigidly flexed, he cured her and the trouble never returned.

WHILE WE ARE ON the subject of the mind, I find this next story – one of mental telepathy – very difficult to explain, and I can only report what I was told by my patient. Mrs Joyce had been

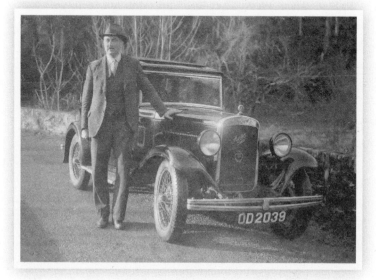

Visiting patients in rural Devon.

in bed with a severe bout of influenza. She still had a trouble-some cough and occasional mild facial neuralgia, but she was a restless soul and being bedridden was an anathema to her, so after four days I allowed her to get up. After not seeing her for a few days, I called on her on a Saturday morning. To my surprise, Mrs Joyce was in bed, looking very agitated and woebegone.

'Whatever is the matter?' I asked her. 'I thought I would find you in the garden, enjoying the sunshine.'

'Oh no,' she replied, 'I have had the most terrible night. I am quite sure that Elizabeth is dead.'

I had not heard her mention an Elizabeth before, so I en-quired who she was and indeed why Mrs Joyce appeared so worried.

'Oh, Elizabeth is my married daughter, and she and her husband Jack live in Singapore. At ten minutes past three this morning I awoke, and there was Elizabeth standing in a luminous light at the end of my bed. For a moment I couldn't move or speak – she just stood there staring, so I switched on the bedside lamp to note the time. As I did so, she vanished. I have just telephoned the post office and sent a cable to Jack to ask if all is well, but I feel certain that Elizabeth came to see me at the moment of her death.'

The next day I telephoned Mrs Joyce to enquire whether she had received any news, but none had come. However, she phoned me on the Monday to report that Jack had cabled, saying that Elizabeth had had to undergo an emergency appen-dectomy, but that the operation had been successful and all was well.

Some months later I noticed Mrs Joyce walking with a young lady on the opposite side of the road. On seeing me, she waved and beckoned me over.

'Oh, Doctor,' she said happily, 'this is my daughter Elizabeth. Do you know, we have compared times and, at the moment she appeared at the foot of my bed, she was actually lying on an operating table, about to be anaesthetized. She says her thoughts were with me at the time, and she wondered if she would survive the operation and ever see me again. Thankfully all is well,' she added with a smile.

I cannot blame Mrs Joyce for reading so much into her vision, as I myself was not above paying undue attention to strange omens! When the post came one morning I was delighted to receive a registered envelope on which was affixed a beautiful set of stamps from the Cayman Islands in the Caribbean. Some of my patients were very thoughtful indeed, and one of them, who was enjoying a world cruise, remembered that I collected stamps and had very kindly thought of me when visiting the islands. Her letter was most interesting; she wrote about the islanders, who were called Caymanas, and explained that their main trade was breeding turtles for turtle soup. Anyway, I put the letter away, and it was completely out of my mind as I attended to my surgery and did a few home visits.

After lunch I read the newspaper and, on turning to the racing pages, the name of the first horse to catch my eye was Caymanas. Well, I thought, this is an omen and I must back this horse.

When I told Nan she said, 'But you know nothing about horseracing, so before throwing your money away, why not phone your patient Mr Blake, who is always backing horses and seems to do well from it, and get his advice.'

This I did, but Mr Blake was not the least bit optimistic. He told me the odds were 33–1 and said that, as he knew nothing of the horse's past, he wouldn't touch it. I didn't heed his advice, and the horse romped home in first position!

A few months later I made a similar wager. A clerical friend of mine was sitting beside me on the sofa in my lounge studying the *Exeter Diocesan Gazette*, and on one of the pages I noticed the names of several of the Devonshire parishes. One I particularly noted was Chudleigh. Now, believe it or not, the name of the first horse that I saw in the paper the following day was Chudleigh. I did not worry about consulting my racing friend this time. I backed it, and it came in a winner at 20–1.

'Your grandfather was our doctor for many years and I owe my life to him, as well as that of my son. As soon as I went into labour, Dr White-Cooper could see there were complications and he whipped me into Dartmouth Hospital where I underwent an emergency Caesarian, which was a very rare procedure in those days. He was a lovely, kind man and a real family doctor!'

PEGGY HAYES, 2012

9

'A Profoundly Difficult Time'

So Much Change in the 1930s

'DOCTOR, I WANT YOU TO CUT MY WRISTS.'

My patient, an elderly lady, had walked into my surgery one morning, sat down and made this extraordinary request. My jaw dropped.

'My dear, if you are contemplating suicide I certainly don't wish to be arrested for your murder,' I replied, eyeing her closely for signs of depression.

'Oh no, I don't mean now,' she smiled. 'Once I am dead. You see, I am terrified of being buried alive – that I should be thought to be dead, but was actually alive. I would bleed, wouldn't I?' she asked.

'Yes, that is correct,' I replied.

'Well then,' she continued, 'I am putting this request in my will, and I hope when I am dead that you will see to it!'

Even after a decade and a half as a GP, my patients still managed to surprise me. I've received many strange requests, but this was certainly a first.

There was also, at around this time, an exciting new treatment for epilepsy that I had an opportunity to try – snake venom. I had paid particular attention to the research because at a young age I developed a fascination with snakes, and in South Africa there are, of course, many species of poisonous snake. These fall into two main categories: those with venom that kills by depressing the brain, causing eventual paralysis of respiration and subsequent death by suffocation; and those with venom that causes rapid clotting of the blood and consequently heart failure.

I was once shown how anti-venom serum is produced. First, the venom was extracted by 'milking' the snake – which entailed getting the snake to bite down onto a piece of rubber pulled tight over a glass jar. Then the extracted venom was injected, in minute drops, into a group of horses (due to their size), and very quickly the horses' antibodies got to work and their blood was harvested for the anti-venom.

Mr F. W. FitzSimmons was at that time a famous snake expert based at Port Elizabeth in South Africa. He considered that minute doses of cobra venom might be effective in the control of excessive stimulation of the brain such as is found in epileptics. Now it so happened that at the time of my learning about this particular medical research I had a young patient who was having as many as four or five epileptic fits per day. I wrote to Mr FitzSimmons and he very kindly sent me a supply of cobra venom, with directions for using it. My patient was treated for some months and, although it did not cure her, the number of daily fits was dramatically reduced.

The venom of the Russell's viper – a Malaysian snake – has been used in suitable weak solution as a styptic, to stop bleeding. It has also been successful in treating uncontrollable nosebleeds and as plugging for a bleeding tooth socket. It stands to reason that these solutions are so diluted that there is no risk of the poison causing systemic symptoms.

It was also around this time that I had the opportunity to put into practice another relatively new treatment that I had once witnessed, a few years back.

A mother brought her seven-year-old daughter to see me one morning. The child had a huge pulsating birthmark over the left carotid region, under her left ear. It measured about 2½ x 1¾ inches. The mother said that she had already consulted two other doctors – one had wanted to freeze it, the other suggested that no treatment was possible. At once I remembered seeing a colleague treat a case at the Hospital for Sick Children in Great Ormond Street, during my time as a house surgeon there. The patient back then had also been a child with a similar condition, and this had been successfully treated with a series of small subcutaneous injections of boiling water to the affected area. When I suggested to the mother that we try the same course of action, she was horrified at the idea and left my surgery quickly, saying that she would like to consult her husband.

Later on, when I explained in detail to the child's father

how these hot-water injections would clot the blood, causing the whole mass of blood vessels to shrink, he agreed to let me treat his daughter. I must say I was a little nervous of carrying out the procedure, although I only intended to inject a small quantity of boiling water.

The child was duly anaesthetized and the injections were given. When I saw the child the following day there was considerable reactionary swelling, and the parents were not too happy. Ice-cold compresses of witch-hazel lotion were applied and within twenty-four hours the swelling had disappeared. The veins, instead of being soft with circulating blood, were now firm and it was obvious the blood had clotted. The girl had two further small injections of boiling water. Within six months the birthmark had completely disappeared, though the skin was slightly darkened over the affected area.

A less-happy first experience occurred after a young man visited my surgery one day, telling me that he had woken up with left-sided earache and could not close his left eyelid. His speech was also slightly slurred and it was clear he was developing facial paralysis – medically known as Bell's palsy. Though not uncommon, I had not seen such a case before. I took a great interest in this young man and felt very sorry for him, for within a few days his whole face was lopsided. Little did I realize that within a month I myself would face a similar plight.

While cleaning my teeth one morning I noticed that the water trickled out of one corner of my mouth, and after breakfast I had some difficulty in drawing from my cigarette. Even then I did not come to consider that I was a candidate for Bell's palsy. What convinced me of my condition was that by tea-time at a patient's house, while eating a sandwich, I could not dislodge food from the right side of my cheek. By the time I returned home I looked a real sight and gave Nan a tremendous shock.

'Oh, Ronald, whatever is the matter with your face?' she exclaimed. 'Could you have had a stroke?'

'Now, my dear, please don't worry,' I told her. 'I am certain it is not a stroke. I believe I may have facial paralysis, possibly caused by a draught through my car window.'

Today it is thought that Bell's palsy is caused by a virus, and in hindsight perhaps I may have caught it from inhaling some of my young patient's breath. Anyway, I fixed a bent hairpin in the corner of my mouth with a rubber band, which went behind my ear, and this tended to keep my mouth straight and make me look a little more presentable, but I must say I was not at all happy about doing my rounds in this manner. Fortunately my condition eased in time, though a slight weakness remains to this day.

I later discovered that my Uncle George also suffered from facial paralysis, which left him with a permanent weakness, although as far as I am aware it is not a hereditary condition.

Another morning, upon waking, I must have got up too quickly, because the whole room felt as if it was revolving, and the floor and ceiling appeared to meet each other. I had developed Ménière's syndrome – a most unpleasant but painless condition, with attacks of giddiness and nausea that come on with no warning at all, and this particular attack lasted some three weeks. I had suffered from mild nerve deafness for some time, and Ménière's syndrome is frequently associated with this.

'COME AND SEE the Leopard Lady . . . the only one in the world. Her mother, when pregnant with her, was once terrorized by a leopard, when she was on holiday in Africa. This is a sight that you should not miss!'

Standing outside a striped tent beating a gong stood a man in a red-and-gold braid uniform that might have made the hall porter at Claridge's green with envy. By the length of the queue, I could see that the Leopard Lady was visibly – and greatly – increasing her bank balance.

I had taken Nan and the children to the Royal Regatta, which was held each year in Dartmouth, at the end of August. During this week there was a variety of activities: boat-racing, sailing, athletic sports, fireworks and, of course, a large fair with its merry-go-rounds, helter-skelter, boxing booths and colourful tents in which you could peer at the world's smallest cow, or the fattest man, or Tom Thumb's brother. However, the Leopard Lady was something completely new to me. I couldn't resist joining the queue.

When at last I entered the tent I saw an intriguing creature seated on a pedestal or throne. She wore a leopard-skin bikini, and nothing else. Having once seen a leopard in South Africa, she certainly resembled one from a distance – her body, apart from her face, was covered in black spots. Everyone seemed

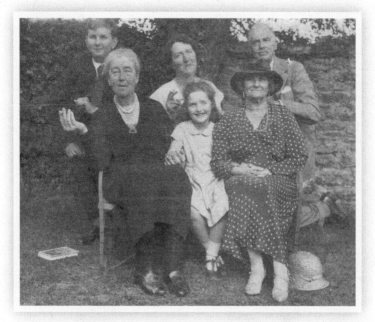

Michael, Cubby, Nan, Althea, my father and my mother.

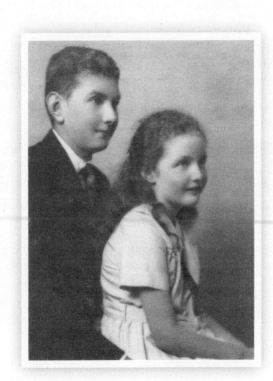

Michael and Althea, 1935.

very curious, peering intently at her once they drew close. As the queue shuffled on, I finally found myself in front of her and was able to whisper in her ear, 'You are a fraud. I know what you do – someone daubs your skin with silver-nitrate solution.'

'Shhhh!' she whispered back. 'My husband does it. No one has ever detected it before. You can have your money back, but please don't tell anyone – you see, it is how I make my living!'

'Well, good luck to you,' I said, 'it is amazing how many fools there are out in the world, and how easily people are taken in.'

The Leopard Lady was, of course, a complete fraud, but the great majority of such freaks of nature are absolutely genuine, and some appear in the *Guinness Book of Records*. At another fair I recall seeing an American lady who was reputed to be the fattest lady in the world. I cannot remember her weight, but it was prodigious, and she could certainly have benefited from a slimming diet; but that seemed the last thing she wanted to do, as weight loss would undoubtedly also have reduced her bank balance. At other fairs I have seen a pony billed as the smallest in the world and a four-legged rooster.

This reminds me of the tragic life of a man named Joseph Merrick. When I was a medical student at St Bartholomew's we learned that he had been nicknamed the 'Elephant Man' on account of his condition, which at the time was thought to be elephantiasis – a disease that causes uncontrolled thickening of the skin and of the underlying tissues. Cast out by society, Merrick was forced to spend many sad years touring all over the continent as a circus freak, until he eventually found his way back to London, where a well-known surgeon, Frederick

Treves, admitted him to the Royal London Hospital in the hope that some surgical procedure might be possible. Eventually it was decided it was inadvisable to operate, but the authorities at the London Hospital felt so sorry for Merrick that they had special accommodation allotted to him. As he was musically inclined, he was also provided with a piano, and one day royalty took tea with him. He spent the rest of his short life living at the hospital – quite contented and in peace – far away from the mocking crowds.

The 'bearded lady' was another fairground attraction one often saw, and I did have two patients over the years who could have earned a living this way, were they so inclined, as both suffered from this unfortunate hirsute condition. One shaved every day, but she was so swarthy that one could detect that she had a five-o'clock shadow. The other had a beard of which many a young man would have been proud. She had three daughters, but none could persuade Mother to shave or use a depilatory cream. A medical colleague of mine was the first surgeon to discover that removal of one of the suprarenal glands would cause this hirsutism to disappear in a few months. On one occasion, when staying with him, he showed me photographs of some fifty women on whom he had operated. The first photograph was taken before the operation, the second about six months later. The difference in their appearance was quite extraordinary. After a few months the excess hair just dropped out. Hirsutism is supposed to be due to a hormonal imbalance and at puberty is sometimes associated with acne.

*

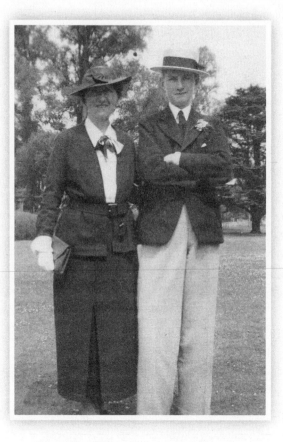

Nan and Michael, Marlborough College, 1935.

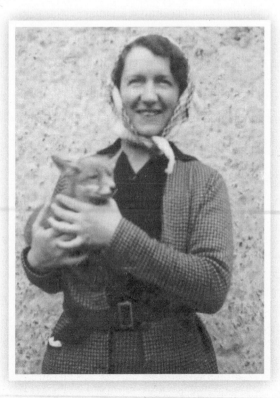

Nan, taken on our last happy family outing –
Windermere, June 1937.

In NOVEMBER 1937 Nan and I decided to take a trip to London. Michael was away at boarding school and Althea and Cubby were visiting cousins in Blackheath so we went to stay at the Cumberland Hotel at Marble Arch.

On 16 November we had been to the theatre to see *Victoria Regina* – a highly acclaimed play about Queen Victoria's reign. On returning to our hotel and after enjoying a light supper, Nan decided to take a bath before retiring. After some considerable time I went to check on her and found the door locked.

'Nan? Nan?' I knocked and called her name, but there was no reply.

I became quite concerned and quickly summoned the hotel staff and the door was broken down. Another doctor was called urgently to the scene, but tragically Nan had suffered heart failure and there was nothing more that could be done. She had died, aged just forty years.

It was a terrible shock for all of us, especially as we were not aware of any weakness. We held her funeral a week later, at St Saviour's, although she is buried in the churchyard at St Clement's Townstal, alongside her younger brother.

As Nan's family had long been living in Dartmouth and she had been keenly involved in the running of social affairs of the parish and interested in the work of the Dartmouth Hospital and the Nursing Association, she knew a great many people and there was a very large turnout for her funeral. I was also very touched to see so many of my patients there, although I suppose by then a number of them had become good friends. Everyone was very kind to our family, but it was a profoundly difficult time. Michael was seventeen and just about to finish his schooling at Marlborough College. Althea, aged ten, was still receiving her lessons at home and I was very pleased that she was not yet away at school, as she was a source of great comfort to me.

Although she was very young, Althea became quite involved in running the house, with the help of our two very good maids: Beryl, who was the daughter of a local farmer; and Doreen, who was in her forties and, according to Althea, had hairs on her chest! There was only ever one serious mishap that I recall, and it occurred soon after Nan passed away. One afternoon Althea went into the kitchen where Doreen was ironing, using a heavy, metal flat-iron that was heated on the wood stove. Usually there were three irons in use on ironing day – one that was being used, one that was reheating and one that was red-hot and ready to go. For some reason Althea went to pick up this last iron, not realizing how hot it was, and the handle stuck to the palm of her hand, burning her quite badly. She managed to shake off the iron and ran screaming out of the house and down to the garden where, outside the greenhouse, she plunged her blistering hand into a tank containing water, blood from the local slaughterhouse and manure from local farms – a mixture that I used for cultivating grapes.

Fortunately, once I had cleaned the wound with surgical spirit and dressed it, it healed remarkably well, with no infection and not even a scar. However, at the time she gave me such a fright, and I was so cross with her, that I paddled her backside with a hairbrush – and I don't think she ever forgot it!

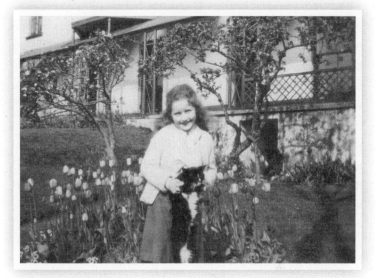

Althea with her cat, George, in the garden at Ridge Hill.

In the months of grieving that followed Nan's sudden passing, I was rather rundown and developed a chronic case of influenza. One of my medical colleagues suggested that I should go on a sea voyage to recoup my health. I wasn't keen on leaving Althea so soon after losing her mother, but thankfully, because of her close relationship with Cubby, she seemed quite content to stay behind. As it happened, this trip away turned out to be a complete fiasco. Ever since the end of the First World War I had been periodically plagued by a duodenal ulcer, aggravated by life at the front and not improved by a daily diet of bully beef and stale biscuits. I more or less managed to control the hunger-like pains with a restricted diet and by drinking an alkali-and-belladonna mixture, and I would go for two or three months without symptoms, and then overwork, worry or some dietary indiscretion would precipitate an attack. However, when I embarked on the Mediterranean cruise my digestive system seemed in good order.

On the second day at sea we were in the Bay of Biscay, which happened to be as calm as the proverbial duck pond, and I was playing a game of deck tennis with a young fellow after a rather large lunch, which included some lobster mayonnaise. It was no doubt foolish to eat lobster, and still more foolish to play deck tennis so soon afterwards, but in the middle of the game I suddenly felt faint and began to perspire heavily. I told my young opponent that I needed to lie down in my cabin, but on the way down I experienced severe abdominal pain and went to one of the lavatories.

The next thing I remember is that I was lying on the floor

of the lavatory, but could not get out because each time I raised myself up to try and turn the latch, I lapsed once more into unconsciousness. I shouted for help, but at 3 p.m. on a Sunday afternoon the stewards were off-duty and most of the passengers were resting.

At last, with what felt like superhuman strength, I managed to free the latch and crawled on all fours to my cabin, leaving a trail of dark blood behind me. I immediately pressed my cabin bell and the ship's doctor was summoned. I told him I was a medical man and had suffered a severe haemorrhage. Unfortunately I was forced to spend the rest of that expensive trip on my back in my bunk. I was never so glad to get home again.

Some months passed with no further discomfort, until one evening I was at the cinema with friends when I began to sweat and noticed my mouth becoming dry. I had no pain, but my heart was pounding and I felt quite faint. I also noticed that my pulse was very rapid. Once again I was undoubtedly bleeding into my bowel. With a duodenal ulcer, haemorrhage is evacuated through the bowel, unlike a gastric ulcer, from which it is vomited.

I had to stay in our local hospital for four weeks, after which I went to London and, on the advice of a specialist, underwent a partial gastrectomy – a procedure that entails the removal of half of the stomach – which meant that I could only take very small amounts of puréed food for a few years thereafter.

There was a most peculiar sequel to this. I had recently been with friends to see the well-known Disney film *Snow*

White and the Seven Dwarfs. On the second day after my operation I was obviously heavily sedated with morphia, when this conversation started.

'Do you believe in fairies?' I asked my nurse.

'No, of course not – there are no such things,' she replied.

'Well, Nurse, you are wrong, because Snow White and the Seven Dwarfs are walking across the end of my bed! I expect you will say I am delirious, but I am as normal and sensible as you. If you wait, I will catch one for you.'

I made several unsuccessful lunges at the little men.

'Doctor, don't be ridiculous. If you keep on doing this you will burst your stitches,' said my nurse crossly.

So I was persuaded to cease my efforts, still absolutely convinced in my own mind that those little dwarfs were solid and alive and walking across my bed. It confirmed to me that people with delirium tremens, or who are delirious from any severe disease, are truly capable of seeing imaginary people or animals in their own minds.

Knowing that I'd be out of commission for some time, I had taken on a locum, who turned out to be a great success. He was young, keen and up-to-date. He intended doing a number of locum positions before setting up as a general practitioner on his own. In the end I was laid up for some months, so he had plenty of time to study. He became so popular, and had such a wonderful ingratiating and suave bedside manner, that there was much wailing and sorrow among the younger set and my elderly lady patients when it was time for him to leave. By the number of cigarette cases, fountain pens, books and sweets he accumulated, he was undoubtedly popular with young and old alike, and I fear many of my patients hoped my illness would be prolonged!

ONE GOOD MEMORY that stands out from what was a very difficult year was my growing friendship with the Reverend Fox. He was an elderly retired parson patient with whom I became very close. He was brilliantly clever – a Doctor of Divinity – who had excelled in all his subjects at Cambridge University. I forget his college, but he was such an interesting man and I always enjoyed our chats. Unfortunately he had been born with the spinal malformation known as spina bifida, and as a consequence he was unable to control his bladder and from birth had always worn a urinary bag strapped to his thigh.

'Do you know, Doctor, that I am psychic?' he said to me one day. 'I have had some extraordinary experiences in my life, and I will tell you about some of them. When I was up at Cambridge there was a large lawn at the front of my college, and on several occasions in the evening I would see a figure resembling a monk walking across it. One could actually see the college building right though him. He always appeared to walk from left to right and would then disappear through the walls. Though I made several enquiries at the time, I do not remember any other undergraduate reporting this unusual happening. But then, you see, I suppose it must be because I am very psychic.

'I used to be a great walker in my younger days,' he went on, 'and would often spend the summer vacation on the continent.

On one occasion I visited Chartres in France, and as I entered the famous cathedral everything felt so familiar to me. I had almost certainly been there before, and yet I had never visited this city in all my life. Perhaps it was a case of reincarnation and I might have lived in Chartres in a previous life – who knows?'

His most intriguing story, however, took place rather closer to home.

'I can tell you about the most extraordinary psychic experience a friend and I had together,' he said one day. 'This was a Cambridge college friend, and we had often been on walking tours together. Well, this particular year, instead of going on the continent, we decided to walk across Bodmin Moor – in those days a very bleak moor. You would walk for miles and miles and never see a soul.

'It was a pleasant sunny morning and we decided we would walk across to Bodmin Town. My friend and I were chatting away when suddenly we heard the sound of a horse galloping up behind us and, as we stepped to the side of the road, the horse and rider flew past us.

'"Look at what he is wearing," said my friend.

'Yes, it was most odd; the rider was wearing a steel helmet and what appeared to be the uniform of a Cromwellian soldier. We could not see his front, but he had what looked like a breastplate on his back and a knapsack slung around his neck. What an extraordinary sight to see in this lonely spot! Well, we walked on and as we came over the brow of a hill, we saw a cyclist pushing his bike along. We stopped him and asked him if there was a fancy-dress fête being held in the district, as we had seen a man ride past in the most unusual uniform. He denied seeing any horse or rider and was ignorant of any fête, but we both remarked that he must have seen a man galloping on horseback, as we had both seen him ride over the brow of this hill. However, the stranger was adamant that he had not seen what we described. Now we were both completely mystified, so we retraced our steps to see if we could see any horse hoof-imprints on the road, but there were none.

'Eventually we arrived in Bodmin Town and decided to call in at an inn and have some bread, cheese and cider. In the course of our conversation with the publican we mentioned our strange experience.

'"So you have seen him too?" said our host. "Every few years on this very day one of Cromwell's despatch riders gallops across the Moor. He was caught by the King's cavaliers and hanged, drawn and quartered here in about 1644."

'The strangest thing about this story,' Reverend Fox added, 'was that both my Cambridge friend and I distinctly heard the sound of the horse galloping up towards us before we actually saw rider and horse go by; and, what is more, we both saw exactly the same uniform. In fact what we described to each other was identical.

'I should have liked to visit Bodmin Moor again on this particular day of the year,' he said wistfully, 'but even if I did, the soldier might not have ridden by, as the publican had explained that this was not an annual event.'

'I was born prematurely in 1934 and your grandfather delivered me safely, rubbed me with olive oil, wrapped me in bandages and cotton wool and put me next to the fire in one of those workers' baskets. You could say it was the first time he saved my life. The second time was six years later when I was ill with pneumonia and a double mastoid infection, and thankfully your grandfather had heard about a new wonder drug which he convinced my mother to give me. Without it, I would probably have died. Your grandfather was a real friend to our family; he looked after us all – even our pet dog Rex. When Rex cut his paw one Sunday and we were unable to get the vet out, your grandfather stitched him up and said to bring him back in a few days so he could check on the wound.

He was a very kind man and I have many fond memories of him.'

JOHN PALMER, 2012

10

'I Want You to Sew
It Back On'

Emergencies and the Outbreak of War

'FOR GOD'S SAKE, Doctor, please come to my house at once!'

I was just going off to my evening surgery when I heard the shout and saw a man running frantically towards me.

'My wife has killed herself – she has swallowed Lysol.'

We rushed to my car and within minutes were at his house. Inside I saw that his wife was unconscious, and between us we carried her to my car, laying her gently on the back seat. Then I made all haste for the local hospital. Here, with great care, I washed out her stomach and gave her all the necessary antidotes.

The following day my patient, Grace, regained consciousness, although she was gravely ill for many days. Cases of Lysol-poisoning are quite rare these days, as Dettol has now replaced this antiseptic. Pure Lysol is a carbolic acid – a deadly poison – and, if ingested, there are only a few cases of recovery. Fortunately this case happened to be one of them.

I found out the cause of Grace's suicide attempt from another patient of mine, who was a particularly close friend of hers. The two women were having tea on the afternoon of the suicide attempt.

'Grace,' said the friend, 'I must tell you something in the strictest confidence. Do you know that your husband has been carrying on for some months with a young girl? I have hesitated to speak to you about it before, but if you don't do something soon, you *will* lose your husband.'

It was a terrible shock to my unsuspecting patient. She burst into tears and her friend accompanied her home, trying her best to calm her. Grace took a little brandy, then said that she would like to go and lie down in her bedroom, and bade farewell to her friend.

I do not know what went through her mind, but she decided to kill herself and to do it in front of her husband. He worked in a local shipyard and returned home from work at about 6 p.m. As he entered the sitting room, he saw his wife standing in front of the fireplace.

'You loathsome beast,' she cried. 'I have heard today that you have been carrying on with another woman for some months – well, you can have her, but you are now also a murderer, as your behaviour will be the cause of my death!'

Whereupon she took a bottle of Lysol from the mantelpiece, removed its top and quickly poured some of its contents down her throat. Within a few seconds she was lying unconscious on the floor. The husband was panic-stricken and absolutely terrified, and ran out immediately to find me.

Grace was able to return home eventually, but the Lysol had burned the lining of her gullet, which had contracted to such an extent that she could only take liquids for the rest of her life. She forgave her husband, as he gave up the girl and became a model spouse, more loving and attentive than he had ever previously been. Perhaps he had learned his lesson?

Another toxic liquid almost caused the death of another patient of mine, but this time it was accidental. A middle-aged lady was having her bath one morning. On the soap dish she happened, very foolishly, to have left an uncorked bottle of Scrubbs ammonia. When stretching forward to pick up a sponge lying across her feet, her elbow knocked the bottle over, causing it to fall into the bath, spilling the liquid ammonia. By a supreme effort she quickly vaulted out of the bath, but not before the ammonia fumes had almost stifled her. She managed to crawl to the bathroom door, which was fortunately open, and shouted for help.

Her cook immediately came to her assistance and dragged her into the bedroom. The effect of the ammonia fumes had apparently caused a temporary spasm of her glottis, for she complained that she had experienced great difficulty in breathing. However, by the time I had reached the house she was breathing normally once again and seemed fairly composed after her ordeal. Had she not vaulted out of the bath immediately, I feel certain her family would have found her dead in the bath from suffocation.

AS OUR FAMILY learned to come to terms with life without Nan, each day in a busy medical practice presented new challenges that left me little time to feel sorry for myself. One young man walked into my surgery clutching a bandaged arm and handed me a brown paper package, in which I found his hand. He was a farm labourer whose hand had been torn off in a threshing machine that morning. The farmer had called me earlier to let me know about the accident, and I told him to apply a tourniquet and to bring the man to my surgery immediately. It was an irregular wound, just above the wrist.

'Please, Doctor, I want you to sew it back on,' the poor man said as he handed me the bag.

Nowadays I believe this might be possible, as there are some wonderful grafting operations being performed, but at the time nothing could be done for the man, except to clean up the wound and create skin flaps, to make a tidy job of the stump. Naturally he went away bitterly disappointed.

On another morning a man walked in with his arm in a sling. He said he had had a fall about a month earlier and had not been able to use his arm since. His wife had rubbed his shoulder with liniment as he thought it was a bad sprain, but when it did not improve he thought it might be wise to see a doctor. I examined him and said, 'Do you know you have been walking about for a month with a dislocated shoulder?'

I tried unsuccessfully to reduce the dislocation and told him to go to hospital early the next morning, when we would reduce it under anaesthetic. When a shoulder is dislocated the head of the humerus bursts its way through the capsule of the joint. We had not bargained for the vent having closed up in the intervening month and, in spite of several efforts by the anaesthetist and me, we were unable to reduce the dislocation. On regaining consciousness the patient was terribly disappointed to hear of our unsuccessful efforts.

'I'm afraid, Mr Jackson, it will mean an operation,' I said. 'We shall have to make a fresh hole in the capsule, then reinsert the head of the bone and resuture the capsule.'

My patient replied, 'If you don't mind, I would like to go away and discuss this proposed operation with my wife.'

'By all means,' I ventured, 'but I am afraid if you wish to make a full recovery and have no further pain, then you *will* need to have this procedure one of these days.'

I did not see Mr Jackson again for several weeks, and then one day he turned up and, on entering my consulting room, threw both his arms in the air.

'What do you think of this, Doc?' he asked gleefully.

Thinking that some other surgeon had convinced him to undergo surgery, I said, 'When did you have the operation?'

'Operation be damned,' he replied. 'I went to see an osteopath. He made me take my coat off, sat me in a chair, walked behind me and got hold of my dislocated arm. He did two or three twists and jerks – mind you, he hurt me all right – but suddenly there was a searing pain, then a click, and then Bob's your uncle, the dislocation was reduced.'

'One up to the osteopath,' I conceded.

Another strange shoulder case involved an elderly man

who came to my surgery complaining of a sharp pain at the top of his left shoulder. On examining him, I felt a hard object like a nail trying to protrude through the skin. I told him I thought it was either a bony spicule or a piece of steel.

'Well,' he said, 'surely it can't be a bit of steel, because how would it have got into my arm?'

'Let's take an X-ray of your shoulder and then we will be certain,' I suggested. Sure enough, the X-ray revealed a thin piece of steel, which I duly removed under local anaesthetic.

The mystery was solved some weeks later when he came to my surgery and said, 'I've been thinking, Doctor, and now I vaguely recall that when I was a boy living in Sheffield, I visited a steel factory and I tripped and fell heavily into a pile of iron filings. What must have happened is that a thin piece of steel entered my arm just above the wrist and over the years has slowly travelled the length of my arm, until it was just about to come out, in the region of my shoulder.'

ON 3 SEPTEMBER 1939, when Prime Minister Neville Chamberlain announced on the radio that Great Britain was once again at war with Germany, he called for calmness and courage. During the opening months of the war, however, the hostilities had very little impact on daily life in rural Devon and, apart from a steady influx of evacuated children from the cities, some of whom became my patients, it was for the most part just a case of carrying on as usual. However, I do remember that there was a real fear that the Germans would drop poison-gas bombs, so every civilian – including children and babies – was issued with a gas mask. We stored our masks in the basement of Montagu, in the children's playroom, which became our air-raid shelter during the war. That was until we discovered that the gas and water mains ran along the side of our house and so, in the event of our house being bombed, we were most likely to be gassed or drowned in our beds. After this, whenever the air-raid siren sounded during the night, we chose to remain in our bedrooms upstairs – and to hell with the Germans!

From 1940, when food rationing was introduced, we were fortunate that our very capable gardener, Hilly, boosted our meagre allowance. He was a wonderful poacher and always wore an old military leather trench coat with huge pockets, in which he kept a pair of rather ferocious ferrets, which he would regularly use to catch rabbits. Often he would give one or two of them to our maid Doreen, who, being a first-rate cook, would roast or casserole them with home-grown vegetables, and we were very grateful for his contribution.

At the outset of the war strict petrol rationing had also been enforced, but thankfully the police and doctors were exempt, which was just as well as one never knew when or where an emergency would arise.

The patients I saw and treated at this time were, by and large, the usual everyday cases of a busy practice. However, one Saturday afternoon I was having tea with a patient friend when the telephone rang. She answered it and then passed the receiver to me, saying, 'It is for you, Doctor.' The caller had apparently phoned my home and been given my patient's telephone number. The voice on the phone said, 'Doctor, please come to the village as soon as possible – there has been an accident on the football field.'

I immediately left my patient's house and fully expected to find a player with a fractured leg or similar injury. However, when I reached the football field I found a young man lying on the ground bleeding profusely from his scalp.

He had apparently headed the ball – a frequent manoeuvre in association football – and the impact of the ball had split his scalp from ear to ear. The wound measured nearly five inches across. It was speedily cleaned out, the hair cut away and the cut sutured, and the young man spent the rest of the game as a spectator, but none the worse for his unusual accident.

Thankfully another unusual head injury also had a happy outcome. I was driving down the High Street one morning when, looking to the side of the road, I saw a baby fall out of its pram onto its head. I stopped the car and dashed to pick up the screaming infant. When the mother hastily emerged from a shop, I told her what had happened. I briefly examined the child's head and there was a good-sized dent in its skull – just as one would see in a dented ping-pong ball. I told the mother to take the child home at once and send for her own doctor, for she was not a patient of mine. She gave me her name and address, and the following day I called in on her – not in a pro-fessional capacity, but just to enquire if the baby was any the worse for the fall.

'Not a bit of it,' she said, 'look at him, he is playing quite happily in his playpen.'

I examined the child's head and the dent had completely disappeared – such is the resilience of an infant's skull. There was no sign of concussion or compression and the child seemed totally recovered from his accident.

FOR MONTHS after war was declared, nothing really seemed to be happening. However, one could not forget that this situation could suddenly change at any time. By 1940 Dartmouth's civic buildings had sprouted sandbags, piled up against their walls to protect them, and there was a blackout at night, with no chink of light allowed to be shown as it might guide an enemy plane.

The impact of the war really started to be felt in early May, with the Germans invading Belgium, Holland and Luxembourg and pushing inexorably towards France. One of my patients – a widow – had an only son, apparently a delightful youth, whom I believe she had always treated abominably. Although she was comfortably off, she supposedly half-starved him and made him sleep in a cold, unhealthy attic. The son was nineteen years old and just about to go to university when the war broke out. Wishing, I suppose, to be free of his mother's clutches, he immediately volunteered and joined an infantry regiment that was sent to France in 1939, to help the French army in the event of a German attack. When the Germans overran France, and British troops retreated to Dunkirk, this unfortunate youth was reported missing, believed killed. The shock of the news caused his mother to collapse and have a complete nervous breakdown, and this is when she became my patient. She castigated herself for the cruel way she had treated her son and vowed never to get out of her bed until she died and joined him. I heard many years later, after I left Dartmouth, that she was still bedridden and was being cared for by her old maid.

After Dunkirk it was thought very possible that the Germans would invade, and as a coastal town Dartmouth would not be safe. In the event of this happening, I made plans to send Althea and Cubby to Dartmoor to stay with friends. I also sent my precious stamp collection away for safekeeping. I carefully packed up my albums in steel boxes and sent them to London to the Chancery Lane safe-deposit vaults, where they were stored underground. Thankfully the invasion never happened, and Althea and her grandmother remained at Montagu, although later that year Althea did leave home to attend Sherborne girls' boarding school in Dorset. (Michael was by now studying theology at Keble College, Oxford.) Since Nan's death, Althea had continued to be a great help with the running of the house and so within a few weeks of her departure, it became apparent that I was in dire need of a housekeeper.

I placed an advertisement in our local newspaper and was quite surprised to receive so many enquiries. Our first housekeeper was a very capable and kind lady in her forties, Miss Dupree. She sometimes had to cope with the unexpected, which she always did most efficiently. It was about 5 p.m. one day and I was at my evening surgery. Meanwhile, at home, the front doorbell rang and Miss Dupree opened the door. To her amazement there stood a bald-headed foreign gentleman – a

Swede, as it turned out – with an enormous fish-hook stuck in his scalp right on the top of his head.

In broken English he explained that he was a visitor to the town and that he had been walking along the river embankment when he saw a number of youths fishing for conger eel. Suddenly he felt a searing pain on the top of his head and realized that one of the youths, casting a hook, had impaled him. The boy cut off the nylon and, leaving the hook in his head, directed him to my house.

Fortunately Miss Dupree was able to escort him to my surgery, where under local anaesthetic I removed the hook, which was nearly two inches long. The Swede was very grateful, and I am sure he will never forget his visit to Dartmouth.

DURING THE WAR some businesses prospered, but not all. Captain and Mrs Drake ran a local business, but things had not been going well and they decided to take in a lodger to boost their small annual income. They put an advertisement in a West Country newspaper, stating that a gentleman lodger would be welcome in a retired army man's household – no children, quiet locality, pleasant garden and otter-hunting in the vicinity. After sifting through a number of applications, they decided on a retired army colonel who had once commanded a regiment on the North-West Frontier in India. Having been in the army himself, Captain Drake was pleased that he and their lodger would have common interests.

Colonel Sharp was also a widower and a teetotaller, and he arrived from London the following week, as he disliked the noise and hustle and bustle of the big city and wanted a quiet country life. He was definitely one of the old-school varieties – a pukka sahib! He had ginger hair and a waxed moustache; yes, he looked every inch the army type. Captain Drake's advertisement sounded perfect for him.

The colonel was a most interesting man, whom I met when asked to dinner one evening. He had seen service in the First World War and had been on several expeditions to Tibet – he seemed the ideal paying guest. He was given a nice large bedroom on the ground floor with a big window overlooking the garden. All went well for several weeks, until one evening after the nine o'clock news, as he and Captain and Mrs Drake were having coffee in the lounge, the colonel suddenly stood up and said, 'I am sorry, but I shall have to leave you tomorrow. I am not used to sitting in a room having coffee with a cow.'

'Whatever are you talking about? Are you joking?' asked Captain Drake.

'No, I am deadly serious!' said the colonel. 'Can't you see that cow behind the piano in the corner?'

'No, Colonel, I think you are imagining it,' said my friend.

'Oh no, I am not,' said the colonel indignantly, 'and, what is more, I think it utterly disgraceful! In fact, it is so disgusting I am going to my bedroom at once. I am not used to farmyard scenes when I drink my nightly coffee.'

The colonel departed in high dudgeon, going straight to his room, whereupon he turned on the light and locked the bedroom door. The Drakes immediately phoned me.

'Please come at once,' they begged. 'Do you remember

Colonel Sharp, whom you met the other night? Well, he's gone out of his mind.'

So I hurried round and we all crept into the garden and watched the colonel through the bedroom window, as he had omitted to draw the curtains. He was charging about the room, knocking pictures off the dressing table, when suddenly he grabbed a tin jug out of the basin and began smashing up the furniture with it, finally hitting the chandelier, so that all the lights went out.

'My friends,' I said, 'I am almost certain your lodger is suffering from severe liquor withdrawal, medically known as delirium tremens, or DTs.'

'But he is a teetotaller,' the Drakes insisted. 'Besides, he has certainly not had a drop of liquor since he has been in this house.'

'That may be so,' I said, 'but occasionally heavy drinkers who have been on the "water-wagon" develop DTs, and the best thing to do is to give them a whisky immediately! However, that's now too late. You must send for the St John Ambulance men or the police, because I will have to give him a powerful injection, and to do that we shall have to break the door down to get at him. He may still have that jug in his hand and clout one of us on the head with it, and then I shall have another patient to attend to.'

A short while later two St John Ambulance men and a policeman arrived on the scene.

'Now,' I said, 'I will get my injection ready, and you fellows must form a battering ram and charge that door. In the meantime, Mrs Drake, will you please hold the torch, so that we can see where the old boy is.'

The four of them lined up one behind the other and went through the door like a tornado. The policeman, being at the front, did a beautiful rugby tackle, and the colonel – jug and all – was on the floor, with the four of them pinning him down. The injection soon fixed him and the St John Ambulance men put him to bed, where I told them he would remain unconscious until the morning.

Having convinced Captain and Mrs Drake that the colonel would not disturb them any further, the policeman and ambulance men departed and my friends and I had a cup of tea.

'Well, the colonel said he was leaving us tomorrow – and he most certainly is, as I will be chucking him out first thing in the morning, but not before he has paid for all the damage he has done,' said Captain Drake.

At about 7 a.m. the next morning there was a light tap on the Drakes' bedroom door and the colonel entered.

'Do you know, my friends,' he said, 'I survived the Quetta earthquake a few years back, but I didn't know you got these things in England. Come downstairs and see my room, it is in a terrible state – a real shambles.'

'Yes,' said Captain Drake, 'and do you know that you were the cause of this earthquake, and you will be leaving us this very day, after paying for all the damage you have done.'

This the colonel did and then meekly left at teatime.

*

By the autumn of 1940, according to my brother Rupert, life in London was very different from that in Dartmouth, with the constant threat of bombing raids. The Blitz had started in September and was decimating parts of the city. A plane dropped bombs over Kingswear in November, but we were fortunate that it was our only raid during that time. While we were spared, the same was not true of my stamps. During the Blitz the vaults at Chancery Lane flooded and my precious stamps, which were all unused sheets, were submerged underwater. When I finally got them back to Dartmouth, they were all stuck together like papier-mâché. It was a most dispiriting sight. However, I had high hopes that I could save them and decided to fill the bath with water and attempt to soak the stamps apart. I'm happy to say that this worked, although we were unable to use the bath for weeks, and there were stamps drying all over the house.

Once the stamps were dry I enlisted the help of Althea and Cubby to paste them onto envelopes addressed to 'The Postmaster, Tristan da Cunha'. I then sent the envelopes (together with some magazines as a gift) to the postmaster there, and in return he franked every stamp 'Tristan da Cunha'. It was such an out-of-the-way place that when all the envelopes returned with that postmark on them, the stamps had doubled their original value. I was delighted, but poor Cubby had lost her glasses – in a bath full of stamps. They were a little clip-on pair and by the time they were fished out they were ruined.

It was probably just as well that Althea left to go to boarding school when she did, because the following year – in May 1941

– her beloved Cubby, who was by now aged about seventy-six, passed away peacefully in her sleep. I remember Althea telling me that she received a letter from Cubby just a day or so after I had rung her to convey the very sad news. Apparently Cubby had written that she was feeling very tired and just wanted to rest. I think Althea felt greatly comforted by the letter, but as she had lost her mother only a few years previously, it was not surprising that she took Cubby's passing very hard. They had been extremely close, and when Althea began her schooling, aged eleven, at Tower House in Townstal, I recall that she would race home each afternoon to see Cubby, and often they would walk in the garden or go out in *The Nancy* – Cubby's rowing boat. It was a clinker-built rowing boat with two sets of rowlocks, where the oars went. Althea was very competent at rowing, thanks to Nan. From the age of eight she and Michael had often accompanied their mother on trips to the mouth of the River Dart to fish for mackerel, which they always delighted in bringing home for dinner.

Alas, a month or so after Cubby's death there was yet more sad news. Althea's nanny, Miss Hearn (or Nanny Minga, as she was affectionately known), also passed away. It was not an easy time for Althea, who was finding settling into her boarding school a challenge. She wrote to tell me that she was often cold and hungry and had befriended the school cook in an attempt to get more meals!

At the end of the year Rupert wrote to tell me that he had rejoined the army as a lieutenant with the Royal Engineers and was being posted to East Africa.

I SUPPOSE IN ONE RESPECT I should be thankful that we did go to war, or I might never have met my future wife and got remarried. It was during the summer of 1941 that I met Alison Mary Arlott, at a hotel in Ilfracombe in north Devon, where I had taken Althea to recuperate after a bad dose of bronchitis. It so happened that Alison, who was tall and blonde and then aged twenty-five, was on holiday with her parents, who were from Surbiton in Surrey. One day we started up a conversation and she told me that she was a trained speech therapist and had worked at two London hospitals, teaching deaf-and-dumb children. I also learned that she had recently ended her engagement to a French gentleman, due to the outbreak of war and various travel restrictions – hence our timely introduction!

A whirlwind courtship followed and about six months later, on 3 February 1942, we married at the Brompton Oratory in Knightsbridge, London. After a celebratory reception at the nearby Rembrandt Hotel, followed by a short honeymoon in Harrogate in Yorkshire, we returned to Montagu. Alison quickly settled into Dartmouth life, getting to know the locals as well as my patients and friends, and within a year she was expecting our first child.

Althea's assertions later on that our housekeeper, Miss Dupree, had rather set her sights on becoming a doctor's wife may well have had a grain of truth about them, as she left us soon after Alison and I returned from Yorkshire. Then Mrs Mock, who was in her sixties and had dyed red hair and an unfortunate limp, took over as our new housekeeper. She too

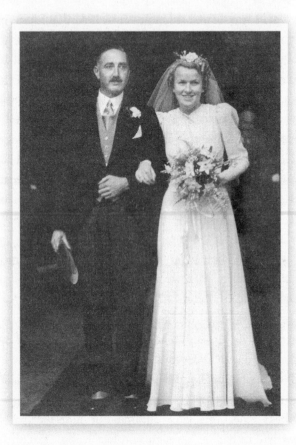

Our wedding day, 3 February 1942.

was very efficient, although not always the most approachable individual.

By 1942 Michael had graduated from Oxford and was based at Oxford House in the East End of London, where he was doing wonderful work in the slums of Bethnal Green. I was not at all surprised at the path he had chosen to follow – he was a good boy and had high principles. He had been very religious as a child, and was never happier than when he was serving as an altar boy at St Saviour's Church in Dartmouth, where his great-grandfather and grandfather had been vicars. At school he had been a rather solitary character but I do recall he became very good friends with the son of the Dean of Canterbury, who he would sometimes bring to Montagu during the holidays.

'I remember Dr White-Cooper but I do not think I was one of the babies he delivered. I was born at Casita Nursing Home in Paignton, as my parents lived in Stoke Fleming. My memories are of a very kind man who, when I was ill, produced chocolate strawberry-creams in foil wrappers. He certainly won a way to my heart! I was quite disgusted that the doctor who replaced him did not give out sweets. I often wondered what happened to your grandfather in Africa. He was well respected by my family.'

JANET BOOTHERSTONE, 2012

11

'A Fatal Ten Minutes'

War Comes to Dartmouth

'DOCTOR, PLEASE COME IMMEDIATELY! PLEASE!'

When I opened the front door after the night bell had rung, what a sight met my eyes! One of our neighbours, Mrs Freeman, was standing there in a nightdress holding a candle, the flame flickering, as her hand was shaking so badly.

She was pleading frantically, 'I think it is my husband in bed beside me, but his face is so swollen I just can't be sure, and he seems to be suffocating!'

I didn't bother to change, but grabbed my medical bag and ran to their house in my pyjamas.

Her husband was a healthy man, so it was shocking to see him sitting on the edge of their bed, cyanosed and making peculiar crowing sounds, as he inspired with great difficulty. He was unable to open his eyes, due to his lids being so enlarged, and his lips were huge.

'Has he been stung by a wasp or a bee?' I asked, opening my bag.

'Yes, as a matter of fact a bee stung him just before he went to sleep last night, but he seemed all right. Is that it, Doctor?'

She told me that she had switched on the bedside light when she heard some extraordinary choking noises, and got such a fright at what she saw. She was absolutely terrified, but fortunately they only lived two houses away from us.

I immediately gave Mr Freeman an adrenalin injection, and within a few minutes he was breathing regularly and his swollen face subsided like a pricked balloon. Within half an hour he appeared perfectly normal.

I had a similar case with a bee sting, and although this patient also had a swelling of the larynx, his face was not swollen. Here again, a subcutaneous injection of adrenalin speedily allayed the symptoms of impaired breathing. A third case was a man who, on swallowing some cider, failed to notice a live wasp swimming in the glass. As he swallowed, the wasp stung him on his palate, which soon swelled up to an alarming size. Once again adrenalin saved him. A bee sting remains in the flesh and contains formic acid, whereas a wasp withdraws its sting, so a bee sting seems to cause more serious allergic symptoms than that of a wasp.

The story of Mr and Mrs Freeman reminds me of another case, but this time the wife's life was saved by the fact that the couple shared a double bed. Mr and Mrs Cunningham were a real-life Darby and Joan. They had no children; there were just the two of them and they lived for each other. They had just celebrated their golden wedding and were already looking forward to the next anniversary. Mr Cunningham, who was recently retired, had been a shipwright at the local shipping yard, where he had been looked upon as *the* man to turn to in the event of an accident, owing to his sound first-aid knowledge and his calm temperament. He was also very thrifty and, on his pension, he and his wife lived a happy life with a host of friends. Now one November night with a temperature near zero they went to bed and, as usual, he put two hot-water bottles in their double bed to warm the sheets before retiring. They had their usual nightcap – a cup of tea – went to bed, turned out the bedside lamp and were soon fast asleep.

In the early hours of the morning Mr Cunningham awoke and, feeling that his feet were wet and cold, his first thought was that one of the hot-water bottles had burst. He switched on the light and, to his horror, found the bedclothes steeped in blood and then saw that his wife was very pale and lying very still. He realized then that one of her varicose veins must have burst and it appeared as though she was slowly bleeding to death.

He quickly put constricting bandages above and below the ruptured blood vessel and elevated the leg. Having desperately tried and failed to wake his wife, who was by this time unconscious, he telephoned me. I rushed over and, with the help of stimulants and warm blankets, she slowly regained consciousness. She was given a blood transfusion the following day. Had Mrs Cunningham slept alone, she would undoubtedly have been found dead in the morning.

DURING THE WAR we Dartmouthians were fortunate in that we were spared the Luftwaffe's nightly air raids, which were devastating many parts of the country – especially considering that the Royal Naval College is based in the town. In fact the college was attacked in a raid in September 1942, resulting in one fatality, but I also remember that Althea could so very nearly have been the second. She was allowed to use the college's swimming pool and was on her way there that day, when the dog she was walking became ill and she (thankfully) decided to return it to its owners, who were patients of mine. One of the town's ship-building yards was also hit that same day and unfortunately there was much loss of life. Many of the survivors suffered very severe wounds, including blinding and loss of limbs. There were six German bombers responsible for the death and destruction that came to the town that day, and though many people believed there were likely to be further attacks, we were certainly not prepared for the 'Tip and Run Raid' a few months later, on 13 February 1943.

The sun was shining and it was a busy market day. Alison was out shopping and I was in my surgery examining a patient with synovitis of the knee joint – it must have been about 11.20 a.m. Suddenly we heard the loud roar of an aeroplane, followed by an angry burst of machine-gun fire. I was sitting at my desk with a large bay window to the side of me.

'Quick, come away from the window, Doctor, it might be dangerous,' warned my patient.

Just as I followed him towards the corner of the room

there was a whistling noise, followed by a loud crash! The bay window exploded with such force that shards of glass pierced the opposite wall. My face would have been cut to shreds, had I not moved in time.

Not so fortunate was the local branch manager of the Midland Bank. He had attended my evening surgery the day before, suffering from acute tonsillitis and a high temperature.

'You will have to spend the weekend in bed,' I told him. 'Get this gargle made up and take these antibiotic tablets every six hours.'

'But, Doctor,' he said, 'I must go down to the bank tomorrow to pay the staff. I shall only be down there ten minutes.'

'All right,' I said, 'but promise me you will return quickly and then go straight to bed.'

'Of course,' he assured me.

Those ten minutes proved fatal. While he was in the bank a bomb was dropped, which completely destroyed the building and killed him, as well as several other people who were inside at the time.

Another patient of mine, who happened to be my tailor, was also killed in the attack. Apparently he told his wife he was just going to the post office and the bank, and he chose the latter first and was there when the bomb fell. Had he gone to the post office first, he might still be alive today – such is fate, unfortunately.

The attack could only have lasted a few minutes, but it was one of many similar assaults causing considerable damage to British coastal towns during the war. Afterwards I was told that at least one of the three raiders in that attack flew in so low that one could actually see the pilot and, instead of coming in from the sea – as one would expect – the plane swooped from behind the town and then soared back out to sea, having dropped its deadly load. Later on, our coastal defence was better prepared and, during another raid, an enemy plane was brought down by anti-aircraft fire.

Altogether some fourteen people lost their lives in this raid on Dartmouth and about thirty were injured. Thankfully Alison was not one of them, despite being caught up in the turmoil. At Dartmouth & Kingswear Hospital my colleagues and I operated on the wounded for some twelve hours.

This devastating attack caused significant damage to the centre of Dartmouth and, to a far lesser extent, the surrounding neighbourhood, including our home and my surgery, though in our case the damage could be repaired. Others were not so fortunate. Considering that Alison was due to be confined a few weeks later, we went to live for a short time in Stoke Fleming – a village some three miles away. A patient of mine had kindly offered us the use of her house: a bungalow on the cliffs. The property benefited from the most spectacular views and the accommodation was most comfortable. However, we did have the strangest next-door neighbour.

She was a Scottish lady from the Western Isles, but the first thing one noticed about her was that she had three rows of eyebrows: two rows on her forehead above her normal one. She told us that on a moonlit night she would patrol the surrounding cliffs with a loaded double-barrelled shotgun in case a German landed from an enemy submarine. I am still unsure as to who would have had the greatest shock!

One day she showed us a cutting from a newspaper to say that the Electricity Commission was considering erecting electric pylons along the cliffs, which she said would detract from the value of her property. I recalled that the renowned playwright George Bernard Shaw frequently spent his holidays in this part of England, so I suggested that she write to him.

'Yes,' she agreed enthusiastically, 'he is bound to cause such an outcry in the press that this pylon idea will soon be abandoned.' This is what she wrote:

Dear Mr Bernard Shaw,
    I know you will be horrified to hear that the Electricity Commission are contemplating erecting a series of telegraph poles and pylons along this part of the coast, at which you have stayed and know so well. We feel it is important for you to write to the press and say how these execrable erections will ruin the beauty spot, then hopefully the project will be abandoned.

Shortly afterwards our Scottish neighbour received this reply:

Dear Madam,
    I love Electric Pylons, don't you?
      Yours faithfully
        G. B. S.

I feel sure that, had Mr Shaw visited this beauty spot at this time, our neighbour might have felt like using her shotgun on him!

THE BIRTH OF OUR SON, William Robert Patrick, on St Patrick's Day – 17 March 1943 – was a very happy event. Alison was attended to by a medical colleague of mine and, thankfully, all was well.

Not all confinements are straightforward, though, and another one at around the same time was certainly peculiar. I received an urgent telephone call to say I was wanted immediately, as there were complications. Fortunately the woman – an evacuee from London – was billeted in a small village nearby. When I got there, I was told that she had gone to the toilet and, while sitting there, her baby had been born. On examining her, I found the baby dangling by its cord in the lavatory pan; luckily its head was uppermost, otherwise it would undoubtedly have drowned. It was a simple matter to sever the cord and help the mother back to bed, where she and her child recovered from this most unusual delivery.

There was another happy family occasion a few months later on 21 September 1943 when Michael, then aged twenty-three, was ordained as a deacon at the parish church of St Nicholas and St Giles in Sidmouth, Devon. Then, the following April, we celebrated his marriage at St Saviour's to a delightful girl – Ann Chinchley Thornton – who was in the Wrens and was the daughter of a Royal Navy commander. The story of their first meeting is a rather amusing one. Long before he began

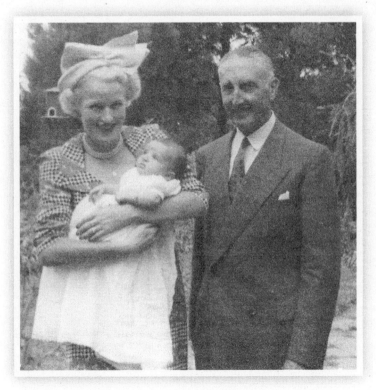

The day of Rob's christening, 1943.

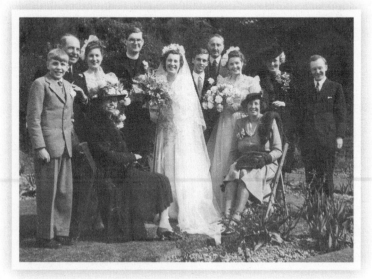

Michael and Ann were married at St Saviour's Church, 1944.

his training for the priesthood, Michael would love nothing more than to potter about in the sacristy at St Saviour's, dressed in his altar server cassock. One day while he was there, Ann approached him, and, presuming him to be the vicar, she asked if he would hear her confession. Michael had to explain that the vicar would be there shortly, but fortunately Ann saw the funny side of it and they became firm friends.

The cherry on the cake for the happy newly-weds came a few months later in September 1944 when Michael was ordained as a priest and just one day later was given his own church – St Francis, Woolbrook, also in Sidmouth. This was a very high honour for someone still so young and I was extremely proud of him, especially when I recall his school days and how desperately he had battled with his studies on account of his being terribly short-sighted. This was only discovered when he was about fifteen years old and thankfully, once he started wearing glasses, he was much happier and his schoolwork improved greatly.

DURING THE WAR Dartmouth was an important centre of naval activity, and the Allied navies made good use of its deep-water harbour. During the latter part of the war the town also became a base for US forces and was one of the departure points for Utah Beach in the D-Day landings. The Americans used Coronation Park – a reclaimed stretch of land situated at the bottom of Ridge Hill, where we lived – to repair the damage to landing ships, sustained during exercises. There were several American commandos stationed about three miles outside the town. They started arriving at the end of 1943 and boosted local businesses – so much so that I sometimes wondered whether our shopkeepers hoped the war would last for years, so that the Americans' stay would be infinitely prolonged.

It so happened that one day an old lady from one of the out-lying villages came in by bus to see me. She was suffering from nephritis – a form of inflammation of the kidneys.

'The next time you come and see me, please bring me a sample of your water, so I can test it,' I told her.

Well, the old lady came to see me again a few days later and, when I requested the specimen, she produced a one-pound note instead.

'You see,' she said, 'I got onto the bus at the second stop and I had the specimen all ready for you. The only bottle I could find at home was a Johnnie Walker one, so that's what I used. Well, several American soldiers got on at the following stop and sat near to me, and then, when the bus got to Dartmouth, they all hurried off again before I could alight. When I put my hand down to pick up the bottle, it was gone, but this pound note was left in exchange.'

'You had better bring in a specimen in a similar bottle each day,' I suggested, 'and you will soon be quite wealthy.'

I only hope those Americans enjoyed that particular brand of Johnnie Walker whisky!

On 3 June 1944 the British and American forces left Dartmouth to invade Normandy. The town was much quieter as a result. The landings were successful and, with the liberation of France, we started to feel that the war would be won. On 8 May

1945 Germany surrendered and the war in Europe at least was over. That summer we were enjoying a rare family holiday in Cornwall and, one glorious day, I had taken Alison and Rob for a beach picnic. Alison was just laying out our lunch from several baskets when a Wall's ice-cream man came by, ringing the bell on his tricycle.

'Oh, Daddy, can I have an ice cream?' asked my youngster.

'No,' I said, 'not before lunch, but I'll tell you what we will do: we will walk along the beach at teatime and I will buy one for you then.'

Satisfied with this answer, Rob sat down and we all tucked into our family lunch.

At about 3.30 p.m. he said, 'Daddy, there is the ice-cream man along the beach, can I have one now?'

About one hundred yards along the beach I could see a collection of some thirty adults and children, so off we went. However, when we arrived at the spot, we found instead a man who appeared to have drowned and who had just been washed up by the sea. People were milling around curiously, perhaps wondering how long the poor man had been dead.

'Come on, we cannot leave him like this,' I said to them quickly. 'We must try artificial respiration.'

I did not mention that I was a doctor, but asked a bystander to lift the man up by his legs to allow the water to run out of his lungs. I then applied artificial respiration by compressing the man's chest, as this was in the days before the vogue for mouth-to-mouth breathing.

As soon as I stopped, I got another man to carry on.

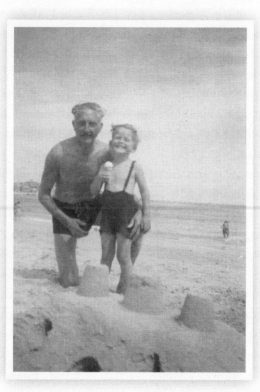

With a very happy Rob and his ice cream, St Ives, 1945.

Fortunately the coast guard had spotted us and soon arrived and offered their services.

'Yes,' I said, 'I want brandy, hot-water bottles and blankets; also an ambulance to take this man to hospital as soon as possible.'

At this stage I had detected a flicker of a pulse and told the onlookers, 'Though he is unconscious, he is not dead, so we must keep up the good work.'

By the time the blankets, brandy and hot-water bottles had arrived and been applied to the man's body and the ambulance had turned up, the man was semi-conscious.

I must admit I was extremely surprised to see that not one person on the beach that day seemed able to carry out an elementary life-saving activity, especially when one considers that first-aid classes had been held all over England during the war.

My family and I returned home the following day. I forgot to ask which hospital the ambulance took the man to, and I never knew his name. What is more, he will never know by what miracle his life was saved: by my young son asking me to go in search of an ice cream!

I HAD TAKEN ON a new locum by now, after some quite mixed experiences in the past. I suppose it is only natural that the cream of the medical profession prefer to work for themselves rather than on another doctor's behalf.

Dr Roberts was an absolute gem. He had plenty of private means, and did locum work for a purpose that I only

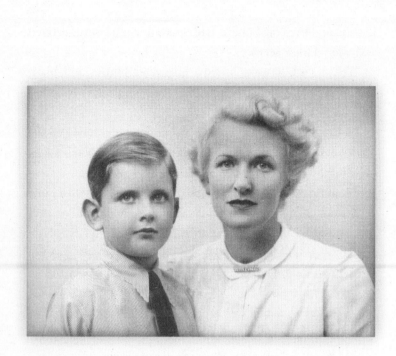

Alison and Rob.

discovered later on. He was a bachelor of about sixty and lived with his elderly mother. I believe he had spent most of his life doing locum jobs in various parts of the country, as he never mentioned that he had been in private practice. Alas, I was on the sick list once again, with a bad bout of influenza. At the end of each day, Dr Roberts would return home and, after the evening meal, he would come into my bedroom to tell me about the day's work. After about the third evening he shook his coat pockets, whereupon there was a loud jangling sound and from them, lo and behold, he produced some George III spoons, a Queen Anne mustard pot and a little silver snuffbox, which he said was at least 200 years old.

'Dr Roberts,' I said, 'tell me, are you working for me or for yourself?'

'Oh, for you, Doctor, of course. But whenever I leave a patient's home I always enquire whether or not they have any old silver they wish to get rid of. I tell them that I collect it and give exceptionally good prices – far higher than they would get at auction. I have a little black book right here in my coat pocket, in which I note the silver marks on all the articles proffered to me,' he added, smiling.

By the time Dr Roberts left me he must have cleaned up the district, for night after night, like a conjurer, he would produce the most wonderful pieces of silver.

'I was born after the war, in 1946, and my mother tells me the story that, while living at 13 South Ford Road, I became very ill with whooping cough. As a bonny baby, I lost a considerable amount of weight as a result of this illness – it nearly killed me – but your grandfather came to the rescue! He was a frequent visitor to our house as my grandmother suffered from kidney disease. I consider it an honour to be quoted in this book.'

MERVYN BROOM, 2012

12

'Such Sadness'

Misdiagnoses and Loss

WHEN I FIRST MET SAM he cut an impressive figure, at about six feet three inches tall. He had recently retired from the London Metropolitan Police and, along with his wife, had moved to Dartmouth. At first he played bowls in the local team, but he soon found visits to the nearby pub more enjoyable and gave up all forms of exercise. He drank such an excess of beer that, at the time of this incident, he must have weighed nearly twenty stone.

Sam also had an evil temper and soon lost one friend after another, gradually becoming more and more depressed.

One morning I received an urgent phone call to go to his home immediately. When I arrived there was a crowd of people huddled around the front door, including his wife, who was looking out anxiously for me.

'Please hurry, Doctor – quick!' she said tearfully. 'Sam is upstairs trying to commit suicide. He's cutting his throat with a razor. Please go and take the razor away from him and stitch him up.'

When I reached the bedroom, Sam was sitting on the bed with blood streaming down the left side of his neck, gripping a straight razor firmly in his hand. He had bloodshot eyes and looked as if he was in the mood to cut my throat, too. I had to get the razor away somehow, before I could deal with him. How was I to do so?

'Hello, Sam old boy, I am sorry to see you've cut yourself shaving!' I said cheerfully.

It was the most absurd remark, but for some reason it worked. Slowly Sam folded up the razor and handed it to me. I threw it down the stairs and went about stitching up the wound. Fortunately he had only cut a small branch of the jugular vein.

A month later his wife called me out again. This time he had made a better job of it and was dead by the time I arrived at the scene.

Cases like this one, where my patient was mentally anguished and, for all my medical training, I could not prevent the outcome, were always distressing. Thankfully they were also quite rare. More common are the number of patients who expect the very worst when they come to see me. It gives me great pleasure to put their minds at rest and send them on their way in a much happier frame of mind.

One day a man came to my surgery with a large swelling over the thyroid gland in his neck.

'You know, Doctor, my neck was normal when I went to bed last night, now look at this enormous lump, the size of a tennis ball – can it be a cancerous growth?'

'No,' I said, 'it is definitely not cancer, or any kind of growth. What happened in the night was that one of the veins supplying the thyroid gland must have burst and the swelling is due to a huge clot of blood, known as a haematoma. I could aspirate the blood.'

My patient did not like the idea of having the blood drawn off by a syringe, but he went away happy, knowing that – though temporarily unsightly – his was not a dangerous condition. I reassured him that, in time, the clot would be completely reabsorbed and his neck would regain its normal shape.

Even more relieved, and surprised, was a cadaverous, pale-faced man with staring eyes who visited my surgery one morning. He sat down and for a moment was quite speechless. Then he said, 'You can do nothing for me. I don't even know why I am here.'

'What's the trouble?' I asked.

'I am dying from cancer,' he said, 'cancer of the throat. I can barely swallow liquids. I have had no solid foods for months.'

'I am sorry to hear that,' I said, 'but it may not be as bad as you think – let's have a look at your throat.'

'It's hopeless. I don't know why I am here,' he lamented again.

With the use of a torch I was able to see an enormous swelling in the region of his right tonsil, which had pushed his palate and uvula over to the right side. The mucous membrane was stretched tightly over the swelling, which was stony and hard to touch, but at one point I noticed a white powdery substance.

'I hope you will allow me to treat you?' I said to him.

'What's the point? I am incurable and dying of cancer,' he said.

I painted the swelling with 2 per cent of cocaine solution and, with a scalpel, made a horizontal incision. With that, a circular white object the size of a golf ball fell out of his mouth onto my surgery carpet.

'There is your cancer,' I said. 'It is a calcified tonsil stone – you haven't a single sign of throat cancer. Go home and eat a juicy steak!'

The man started to weep and put his arms around my shoulders.

'I can't believe it, I can't believe it,' he cried. 'I am not going to die after all.'

'Hopefully not for many years,' I reassured him. 'But before you go, let me get a little box.'

In the box I placed some cotton wool and then the tonsil stone. I don't remember ever seeing a patient leave my surgery in such a happy mood. I never saw him again and hope his future was a bright and happy one.

A MEDICAL COLLEAGUE of mine once related this strange story to me. He was lunching at a small inn, in the dining room patronized by commercial travellers. Seated next to him was a loquacious gentleman, who, not knowing that my friend was a doctor, got onto the subject of health.

'Do you know,' he said, 'a funny thing happened to me about three years ago. I began to find my tongue getting stiffer and stiffer every day – it wasn't actually painful, but made talking and swallowing difficult. One morning I looked at my tongue in a mirror and saw a small lump near the tip. It felt hard. I thought I had better see my doctor. He said he didn't like the look of it, and gave me a mouthwash and told me to see him again in a week.

'Well, the lump got no smaller, so he said I had better see a Harley Street specialist – a great man on tongues. This surgeon looked at my tongue, dabbed it with blotting paper, looked at it again, dabbed it once more and then felt it.

'"I am sorry to tell you, but you have cancer of the tongue," he said.

'Well, you can imagine I didn't like the sound of that, but the specialist went on to say that he would ring up his nursing home and get me a bed immediately, so that he could remove my tongue the following morning.

'"Well," I said, "if you don't mind, I would rather discuss the matter with my own doctor and my wife first, and then perhaps get another opinion."

'"You will be wasting your time," said the great tongue specialist. "You will die if your tongue is not removed quickly, but I will tell you what I will do. I will get in touch with three other tongue specialists I know and see if they agree with my diagnosis, but I'm afraid it is likely you will lose your tongue."

'So the great tongue specialist phoned his three tongue-specialist friends and arranged for them to examine me at

5.30 p.m. the next day. I must say I felt rather honoured that four of the greatest tongue specialists in England were going to look at my tongue. One after the other blotted and inspected, blotted and felt it. Then blotted and felt it once more, after which treatment my tongue was really quite tender! Now the first tongue specialist said: "We are going to discuss your case in another room, after which we will give you our verdict." I felt like a prisoner who had committed murder, waiting for the jury's verdict.

'After about quarter of an hour, the four specialists emerged, looking more like four undertakers. "We are afraid that we are all of the same opinion: that you have cancer of the tongue and that you are going to have to lose it."

'I said, "I am very obliged to you for the interest you have shown in my case, but I would still like to discuss the matter with my wife and family doctor and will let you know what I decide."

'When I saw my home doctor again he said, "If you don't mind, I would like you to see one more specialist – a brilliant man who is a specialist physician, not a surgeon."

'So to the latter I went in desperation. He also dabbed my tongue with blotting paper, looked at it, pinched it and said, "I think I can cure your problem in about a fortnight."

'"You mean to say I will not have to have my tongue cut out?"

'"Certainly not," he replied. "I wish you to take this medicine three times a day and report back in a fortnight."

'Believe it or not, in a fortnight the lump had completely

disappeared. When I saw the physician again I considered him a wizard. "Didn't I have cancer then?"

"'No," said the physician, "your trouble was due to syphilis! It is an unusual place to have it – can you account for it?"

'I remembered then that a friend of mine had syphilis and we frequently played billiards together. We both smoked pipes, and one evening while we were playing I took up his pipe by mistake, and that is probably how I caught the disease. I never saw the four great tongue specialists again, and they must have wondered what had become of me. I expect they are all dead today, but I have never felt fitter!'

IT WAS ABOUT 10 p.m. one evening and I was listening to the radio upstairs, when I heard a loud knock at the front door. As our housekeeper was off duty, Alison went to see who it was and in walked a couple, in a very agitated state. Alison showed them into the drawing room, where they sat down, and she then came to call me. When I entered the room the young woman jumped up.

'Oh, Doctor . . . thank goodness,' she said. 'Frank and I are engaged to be married, but he has just spat up blood, and that means TB, and I couldn't possibly marry a man with TB – it would mean nursing him for the rest of his life.'

What a heartless girl, I thought.

This couple, I was told, had apparently been walking along one of the town's pavements and, as they passed under a lamp post, the young man had spat up something onto a paving stone. To their dismay, they both saw blood.

'Oh, Frank,' the women had said, 'you know what that means – TB. You must come and see the doctor at once. We may even have to break off our engagement.'

The young man remonstrated, 'I am quite sure I haven't got consumption. I would have a cough and would have lost weight, and I have no cough and my weight is quite steady.'

Nevertheless his fiancée was adamant, and that is how they came to be in my sitting room.

Well, I made the most thorough examination, tested the young man's temperature, which was normal, sounded his chest, examined his abdomen and finally looked down his throat. There, beside a lower molar, was a piece of inflamed gum, which was bleeding freely.

'You haven't a sign of TB; in fact you are a particularly healthy young man,' I said. 'All you need is a visit to your dentist. Your teeth could be in a better state, and the cause of your trouble is a bleeding gum!'

I hope the marriage turned out to be a success.

We held our own family wedding celebration a few months later, on a summer's day in August 1946. In a time-honoured family tradition, Althea was married to Richard Rainald Tebbutt at St Saviour's Church. Michael officiated alongside the Rev. Watkins, and as Althea left the church, Rob gave her a lucky silver horseshoe. The church was full to bursting and after the ceremony colourful guests in hats and gowns, top hats and morning coats made their way in the warm sunshine to the reception, which we held in a large marquee at Montagu. The happy couple had first become acquainted at the Royal

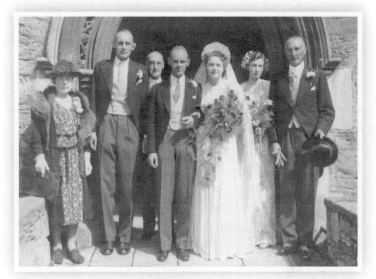

Althea's wedding day, 1946.

Navy's Yeovilton Fleet Arm Station near Somerset in 1944 where Richard – or 'Tim', as he was known – was serving as a senior pilot, and Althea, then aged seventeen, was training to be an Aircraft Direction Wren. In fact their first meeting had occurred on a radar screen! Apparently, Tim (or Caveman Dog, as his call sign was) had been about to fly directly into a range of hills, due to bad weather and poor visibility, and Althea had quickly radioed him to warn him of the danger ahead. He had liked the sound of her voice – as she did his – and when, a few days later, he came to thank her in person, that was that!

THE TOWN'S ANNUAL Royal Regatta and Fair was not held during the war, so there was much excitement in the town as plans and preparations got under way once more for the week-long festivities in August 1946. However, it was not all good news. Over the years I had witnessed a number of tricksters, charlatans and quacks of various kinds who would descend on our town and, having robbed the innocent and gullible, would be gone the following day, never to return.

One day I noticed a large crowd around a lorry. On the back of this lorry stood a youth with a naked chest; and a man, probably his father, was mapping out the lungs and heart with coloured chalks. He certainly knew his anatomy. Having produced the necessary crowd of onlookers, he then began preaching about his various miraculous herbal remedies, which would cure everything from housemaid's knee to bronchitis, not forgetting such common skin complaints as eczema.

He then proceeded to take up a bottle and a test-tube into which he poured a reddish fluid, which he said was urine from a woman suffering from kidney disease.

'Now,' he said, 'you must all watch this very carefully – just two drops of this specific mixed with this urine will dissolve the blood completely.' And so it did. The liquid in the test-tube became clear. (Of one thing I am certain – that red colour was not due to blood.) 'Isn't it wonderful?' he enthused, and the congregated people agreed as one man.

'Now,' he went on, 'when you pass bloody water, it means you have a terrible inflammation in your kidneys. A few drops of my specific, taken three times a day, will cure your kidney trouble within a few days.'

He then produced some medieval-looking surgical instruments, which I think, from the appearance of them, he must have borrowed from a veterinary surgeon.

'Now,' he said, 'how would you like your bowels to be held by these terrible clamps? Yes, this is what surgeons do when they take out your appendix. At the first sign of appendicitis, you must take this anti-appendix draught' – pointing to a bottle with a white liquid – 'and then you won't have to be cut open and pay an enormous surgeon's bill.'

One of my patients, seeing me in the audience, came up to me and asked, 'Getting some useful tips, Doc?'

'Yes,' I laughed, 'isn't it wonderful what the gift of the gab can do!'

Well, before this gentleman had packed up his miraculous pills and potions he had done a very profitable trade with the local population, and I hope they benefited. There was, however, one real tragedy, where a quack was concerned.

I had a young patient, a young man of eighteen, suffering from tuberculosis of the right hip. As was the vogue in those days, complete immobilization of the joint was advocated, as well as taking cod-liver oil and lots of fresh air by an open window. Well, it so happened that I departed on a month's holiday and, in my absence, instead of calling upon my locum, the family was persuaded to call upon an unqualified quack who called himself a 'consumption expert'. The youth was removed to the house of the 'expert' in a neighbouring town and the parents were told that keeping the hip joint immobilized would entail a stiff hip joint for life.

'Your son must have active moments,' claimed the quack, which he duly carried out. However, by doing this he broke down adhesions in the hip joint and liberated countless thousands of tubercular bacilli into the poor boy's bloodstream. As a result he developed acute military tuberculosis and, on my return from holiday, I was told he had died a few days previously.

TOWARDS THE END of 1946 we received some very good news. Michael had been appointed curate at St Michael and All Angels in Brighton, where he rapidly became noted for his eloquent sermons.

According to the letters he wrote me, it hadn't taken him and Ann long to feel at home, as they busied themselves getting to know members of their congregation. Everything seemed

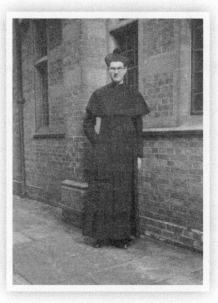

Michael, Curate at St Michael and All Angels,
Brighton, 1946.

to have fallen into place for them and they seemed very happy. Who could have known that such sadness lay ahead? In the early hours of Sunday, 18 May 1947 – Ascension Day – Michael, aged just twenty-seven, suffered a heart attack and passed away. It was a truly terrible time, not least for Ann who also lost the child she was carrying.

Following a celebration of three requiem Masses at Dartmouth, Sidmouth and Brighton, Michael was buried in the churchyard of St Clement's Townstal in Dartmouth, alongside his mother, uncle and grandmother.

After his death I was very touched when a small book of his sermons was published, entitled *The Face of Jesus Christ*. The foreword to the book was written by the Rev. Canon Eric Abbott, who later on became Dean of Westminster. Some of his words held particular meaning for me:

> Michael's . . . sermons breathe the spirit of detachment from the world, as though he intuitively knew that he would himself follow Jesus in dying young. So one of our priests left us when he was yet young. There are ways of sacrifice. One makes the sacrifice of early death. Another makes the sacrifice of a long life on earth. But the real thing is to come to the measure of the stature of the fullness of Christ and to understand that a man feels the advance of his age more by the strengthening of his soul than by the weakness of his body. Thus holiness and only holiness is the mark of Christian age.

At the time of Michael's passing I supposed he must have inherited the family heart weakness that had also claimed his mother's life. However, later on I did wonder if it was a case of undiagnosed diphtheria, as he did complain of a very sore throat in the days leading up to his death. As a vaccination programme for the disease was only introduced in 1940, it is entirely possible that he was never inoculated. If only it had been a few years earlier, this tragedy may well have been prevented.

'I have been a patient [of Dr White-Cooper's] for 27 years and I, like many others, can pay testimony to his patience, sympathy and ability . . . we are losing a doctor and a friend, and I know many would join me in wishing him god-speed as he leaves us.'

Quoted from a letter by MRS LLOYD to the
Dartmouth Chronicle & South Hams Gazette, 1949

13

'I'm Entitled to These for Free,
Aren't I?'

The Birth of the NHS

IN 1948 HEALTH SECRETARY ANEURIN BEVAN introduced
the National Health Service to Great Britain, and everyone was
entitled to free medical treatment. Of course people had to
make a monetary contribution to the service, yet at the same
time they strongly believed they were getting something for
nothing – even requesting small items such as cotton wool,
bandages and lint. It was not long before doctors noticed
how their waiting rooms overflowed; how patients would be
standing in the passage, or even queuing outside in the street.
During that first year I remember prescribing more glasses for
failing vision, and more dentures, than in all the thirty years I
had been in practice in the town.

I particularly recollect one cold, wintry November morning. It had been snowing during the night and the town was

carpeted with a white mantle of snow. A little grey-haired old lady shuffled into my consulting room.

'Good morning, and what can I do for you?' I asked – my customary greeting.

'Oh no, Doctor, I am not ill,' she replied quickly. 'I have just come to get a packet of corn plasters from you.'

'Now come along, Mrs McCreedy, you can get those at the chemist for about a shilling. Surely you don't need to take up a busy doctor's time with such a trivial request?'

'Oh yes, I know,' she said, 'but I am entitled to these for free, aren't I, so why shouldn't you give them to me?'

There was no argument to be had with her.

'I have had a lovely morning in your waiting room,' she went on cheerfully. 'The fire has made it nice and warm, and I have enjoyed reading all your illustrated papers. And of course I have had a good gossip with some of my friends. We were all just saying how much cosier it is in your waiting room, looking at the papers, than in the local library, where there isn't even a fire to keep you warm!'

On another occasion I was called to a patient's home and, on entering the house, saw a group of women sitting around a table stuffing cushion covers with cotton wool.

'Oh look, Doctor,' one remarked, 'isn't it wonderful – all this cotton wool from the surgery, with nothing at all to pay.'

Needless to say, I was once again rendered speechless.

I must say I did feel rather sorry for some of my private patients. Many of them still wished to be treated privately and would say, 'If I am not on your NHS list and you give me a private prescription, I shall have to pay the chemist, and yet at the same time the government gets my contribution.' This especially applied to those who had to have frequent liver injections, cortisone, antibiotics and other expensive drugs.

So gradually my private patients drifted onto our National Health Service lists and only a very small percentage remained as private cases. One of these was a new patient, a senior naval officer who was now retired. For some years he had apparently been treated for cancer of the prostate with large doses of female hormone – the recognized non-operative treatment. He was suffering from acute bronchitis, but seemed diffident about allowing me to examine his chest.

'Is it really necessary?' he asked, folding his arms protectively.

'Yes,' I replied. 'I want to make sure you have nothing more serious – for instance, pneumonia.'

When he finally removed his pyjama jacket, I saw at once that he had a pair of bosoms that a Hollywood film star would have envied! This was of course due to the feminizing effect of the hormones he had been taking to control his prostate growth. He did have a good sense of humour, though, for he joked, 'I suppose that if any of my friends at the Admiralty could see me now, they would probably want to sleep with me, wouldn't they?'

MY FIRST IMPRESSIONS of the National Health Service were not entirely favourable and, after much deliberation, Alison and

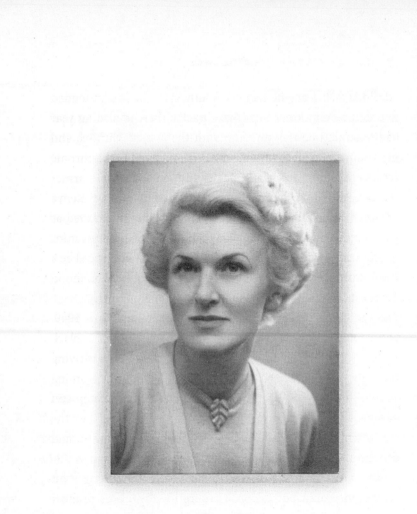

Alison, 1948.

I decided that we would move to South Africa, where I intended to continue my career in private practice. The preceding year had been particularly difficult, with the loss of Michael, and my young son Rob had for some time suffered from chronic asthma, a condition that I felt would benefit from a warmer climate. Althea and her husband Tim had emigrated to Kenya in late 1947, settling in Nairobi, where Tim was employed as an electrical engineer and Althea worked as a census officer for the Kenyan government. Our move to South Africa would be a fresh start in a country of which I had many happy childhood memories.

Our preparations were almost complete by June 1949, and I took Alison off to Torquay for the day. I drove a black Austin 7 at the time and we were on our way home, driving through Kingswear, when I saw a brewer's lorry coming straight towards us. The driver was going too fast to stop and so I pulled the car over as far as I could, into the hedge by the side of the road. He slammed into us with a loud crash – and drove on, disappearing round the bend in the road.

By some miracle it was the rear of the car that was hit (and badly damaged) and not the front, where Alison and I were sitting. We were shocked into silence and very shaken. The police were called – and found the car's rear-door handle twenty-five yards down the road.

We had to appear as witnesses at Brixham police court in July. The driver denied he had been speeding and insisted that he was going no faster than twenty-five miles an hour. To us, it seemed much more like forty! He was found guilty and fined six pounds for reckless driving, and four pounds for failing to stop after an accident.

By then I had ceased practising, Montagu was sold and our furniture packed up so we were staying at the Norton Park Hotel. One of my last duties was to act as judge at a baby show being held as part of the Dartmouth sports carnival. As anyone who has judged a baby show knows, this can be quite a daunting task.

'You cannot please all the mothers,' I said, before handing out the first prize. 'Perhaps it is just as well I am going away.'

Although they smiled politely, I feared that some of the women looking at me certainly agreed.

I was extremely touched by the goodwill and generosity of my patients – from Dartmouth and beyond – many of whom had, over the years, become close family friends and were very sad to see us go, as is shown in the following passages, which are reproduced by kind permission of the *Dartmouth Chronicle & South Hams Gazette*:

Village Farewell to Doctor, July 1949

Patients of 30 Years Ago

Parishioners and friends from the neighbourhood met in Stoke Fleming Parish Hall on Friday to make a presentation to Dr W. R. White-Cooper on the eve of his departure for South Africa after 30 years of ministering to the sick in the village.

During this period many friendships were formed

between the doctor and his patients, and none was more sincere than that between him and the Dure family. As soon as his impending departure was known, Mrs D. Dure concerned herself with arranging a subscription list with the aim of giving Dr White-Cooper some token of their affection and esteem. The gathering was the outcome of Mrs Dure's idea.

The evening opened with a whist drive at which there were 16 tables, the proceeds being ear-marked for the funds of the proposed village playing field. Mr Jack Bowden officiated and on behalf of Mrs Dure he welcomed Dr and Mrs White-Cooper. The occasion, he said, was one of pleasure and regret, more especially the latter, since this was probably the last visit Dr White-Cooper would make to Stoke Fleming.

He paid a very warm tribute to the doctor for the great kindness and understanding he had always shown to his Stoke Fleming patients, and in this connection he could speak from personal experience. If further proof of this was required, the number of people present would afford it, the large majority knowing the doctor both professionally and socially.

They could find some small measure of consolation in the fact that their loss would be someone else's gain, and whatever the future might hold for Dr White-Cooper and his family, Mr Bowden ended, they could be assured of the best of good wishes from Stoke Fleming.

First Patients

Mr Bowden asked the doctor to accept a token of their esteem from a group of some of his first patients in the village. Dr and Mrs White-Cooper were escorted to the stage to the accompaniment of hearty applause. The presentation was a magnificent three-branch silver candelabra – a truly exquisite example of the silver-smith's art. The doctor also received a 'biro' pen.

Speaking under obvious emotion Dr White-Cooper thanked Mrs Dure personally, and the village as a whole, for the quite unexpected present. He recalled his early days in Dartmouth and Stoke Fleming and said he wondered, on his first visit to the village and when no patients were forthcoming, whether he would have to apply for admission to the Totnes Institution! However, aches and pains made their appearance in due course and he was thereby saved from having recourse to such a step.

Honest Friendship

He said that it would be quite impossible for him sufficiently to thank his Stoke Fleming friends for their confidence and fellowship during the years he had been in attendance in the village and he would ever remember the kindness everyone had shown him. He gladly accepted the truly beautiful gift, in the spirit in which it was given him – honest friendship. It would be a lasting reminder of the happy (and, unfortunately, sometimes not too happy) times he had spent in Stoke Fleming.

Doctor's Thanks

Dartmouth Chronicle, 14 July 1949

Sir,

May I, through the courtesy of the *Chronicle*, convey my most sincere thanks to all my patients and friends for the many messages of goodwill sent to me on the eve of my departure from Dartmouth. I have received many letters conveying good wishes, and last week, at the Baby Show during the Dartmouth Carnival, I was deeply touched when I was presented with a lovely sealskin wallet containing notes.

I would like to say thank you to all. I shall carry with me on my travels many happy memories of the 30 years I have spent in Dartmouth, and some sad ones too, but through them all the kindness and friendliness of everyone has been outstanding.

My wife, my son Robert and I will not say goodbye, but only *au revoir*, and we send our best wishes to you all.

Yours, etc.,

W. R. White-Cooper

14

'Honey, Water and Faith'

A New Start in South Africa

IN SEPTEMBER 1949 my family and I sailed into Port Elizabeth harbour, intending to settle in the town, mainly because of its proximity to Grahamstown, where I was born. However, it was not as we expected, and so we began to look elsewhere. I had previously been asked to represent the British Medical Association at the Commonwealth Medical Conference that was being held in Cape Town later that month. As we motored down the Garden Route to Cape Town, we happened upon the town of Somerset West, situated at the foot of the Helderberg mountains and nature reserve – surrounded by orchards, farmlands and vineyards. We were immediately captivated by the area's great beauty and it was here that we decided to make our home.

After spending the first two months in a small residential

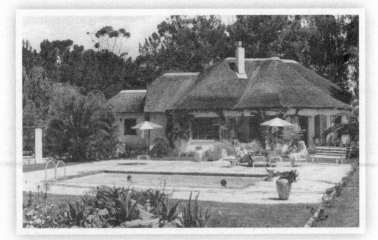

Fulmer Lodge, Somerset West.

hotel, we eventually found an ideal house – a thatched bunga-low with two and a half acres of garden and numerous fruit trees, which we named Fulmer Lodge, after the Buckingham-shire village where my paternal grandparents had once lived. The owner was emigrating and we were able to take over his cook, who lived on the property and whom he assured us was honest, reliable and excellent.

For months, Fred – the cook – was most satisfactory and we congratulated ourselves on our good fortune. Then one morning Alison went into the kitchen to go through the day's menu with him. As she entered the room she noticed a most peculiar odour, but thought no more about it. Fred appeared to be in a particularly good mood, perhaps even a little more loquacious than usual. After giving him his instructions, Alison went to telephone a friend and then sat down to read the *Cape Times*. As she was reading the paper she became aware of peculiar sounds coming from the kitchen.

Suddenly Fred rushed into the lounge, his eyes bloodshot, a terrible grimace on his face, with both hands outstretched towards her. He was squealing and making the most uncouth sounds, evidently intent on harming her. Alison jumped out of her chair and fortunately got to the front door before Fred could reach her. He proceeded to chase her across our lawn, but then suddenly fell down, appearing to have some sort of seizure. Alison was beside herself with fear and could barely speak when she telephoned me at the surgery, and I rushed home immediately. Fred was lying unconscious on the lawn, so I called an ambulance and got him admitted to our local hospital.

Unbeknown to us, that morning Fred had been smoking marijuana – or dagga, as it is known locally. Once he had recovered, I explained to him that as he had suffered a fit, he should not continue to work as a cook as it was possible that he could have another seizure while cooking, and injure himself.

'So, Fred,' I told him, 'I am afraid you will have to leave us and look for another position.'

Believe it or not, a fortnight after being discharged from hospital we heard that Fred was in the local gaol, having stabbed a man to death. He was tried and sentenced to just eighteen months' imprisonment. I was staggered at the light sentence, but apparently the man whom Fred had stabbed to death had gone off with Fred's girlfriend while he was recovering in hospital, and in view of this the judge had exercised leniency.

The story continues some eighteen months later, when Alison returned home from shopping, looking quite pale and shaky.

'Whatever is the matter?' I asked her.

'Oh, I have just seen Fred in town. He is obviously out of gaol, and I'm sure he will come back here and try to murder us,' she replied.

'Why should he? We've done him no harm,' I said.

Well, just a few days later Fred did indeed turn up at my surgery, all smiles, saying how pleased he was to see me again and could I please give him a reference? Needless to say, a reference was not forthcoming.

*

NOT LONG AFTER we had settled in Somerset West I was invited to join a busy medical practice on Main Street, with two other local doctors, one of whom I had known well from my days as a GP in Devon. Of course among my first few patients I saw and treated were many of the same ailments and illnesses that I had seen in Devon, but I also had to familiarize myself quickly with the symptoms and treatments for some new and potentially life-threatening situations. Now, as well as dealing with bee stings, I had to look out for the bite of the South African button spider, which produces a venom just as deadly as that of the cobra or mamba snake. Because of the minute quantity of venom injected, I learned that the bite was unlikely to prove fatal to a healthy adult, but could kill a child.

I also discovered that I had much to learn about a certain kind of patient whom I had never encountered in England. Perhaps I had been lucky, but as this story will show, I was consequently rather naive.

After living in Somerset West for a few months I had become friendly with the local physiotherapist, and on several occasions he sent me new patients. One evening he came to my house and said to me, 'I have just seen a middle-aged lady this afternoon who is down here on a holiday from Rhodesia. She seemed rather breathless, and I noticed her legs were rather swollen. She had come to me for a massage. I told her, "I don't think you need to see me. I suggest that you take yourself to bed, and I will send a doctor to see you in the morning."'

That is how I came into the picture.

The patient, Mrs Gold, was a rather stout woman. She and

her lady companion were both Jewish, and I presumed they were Orthodox, as they both wore very obvious wigs. Mrs Gold had a dilated heart and I prescribed appropriate treatment and bed rest. She said she had come to Cape Town because her husband, who suffered from diabetes, had to go into a nursing home to have two toes amputated for diabetic gangrene. She told me that he was a cattle rancher from Rhodesia, and that another reason for her visit was to find a new manager for their ranch.

One day I called to check on her and found her examining a large number of cheques, which were laid out all over her bed. Each was made out to her and was for an identical amount.

'Oh,' she explained, 'you see I put an advert in the local paper offering a very large salary for a ranch manager. Applicants had to write in with their qualifications and send a deposit of ten pounds.'

How many of these cheques were ever returned to the unsuccessful applicants I shall never know, but Mrs Gold went on to tell me that she had a son who was studying economics at Oxford University and then showed me his photograph. He certainly bore no resemblance to his mother. 'He's the very image of his father,' my patient assured me.

Well, Mrs Gold definitely seemed to be getting stronger and so I allowed her up for longer each day. One morning on the table by her bed I noticed a book entitled *The Diabetic Life* by Dr R. D. Lawrence.

'Whatever is this?' I enquired.

'Oh, that's for Daddy, when he returns from the nursing

home. He must have a special diet, and this book will tell me how to feed him.'

On another visit Mrs Gold showed me a cable that she had received from the Standard Bank in London, which told her that a bank draft for £10,000 was being sent to her local bank. This cable was also shown to a number of shops in the vicinity by Mrs Gold's companion and, of course, after this Mrs Gold was allowed as much credit as she liked by one and all.

One evening my friend the physiotherapist came over and told me, 'I have just heard that Mrs Gold's son – the one at Oxford University – has been killed in a motor-car accident as he was driving back from Epsom after seeing the Derby.'

Well, you can imagine that, knowing of my patient's weak heart, I immediately telephoned the house where she was staying. Her friend told me that Mrs Gold was naturally greatly shocked, but that she had given her a brandy and some smelling salts, and that Mrs Gold was now sleeping and I was to call round in the morning.

When I arrived at the house, before my morning surgery, there was a notice pinned to the door on which was written: 'Gone to Cape Town to see Daddy.' I thought it only natural that she had gone to break the sad news to her husband and gave it no further thought as I attended to my other patients. Unfortunately I was unable to visit her again during the day as a confinement case kept me busy, but when I spoke to her companion later on, I was told that although Mrs Gold was still broken-hearted, I could come and see her the following morning. This I did, but to my surprise when I arrived at the house I found about a dozen people milling around and peering through the windows into the house. One very upset man explained that the ladies had left the district in the dead of night, and that he and the other people waiting outside the house were some of their trusting creditors!

Well, I phoned up every nursing home in Cape Town, but none of them had ever heard of Mr Gold. Subsequently a police investigation revealed that not only had Mrs Gold no son, but that she had never married, and that she and her companion were wanted for fraud in several towns in South Africa – in fact they were the country's most infamous female criminals at the time. There was no cattle ranch; the cable from the Standard Bank was phoney and was probably sent by an accomplice in London; and the diabetic book was bought purely to impress me.

Some weeks later Mrs Gold and her companion, dressed as men, were arrested at Cape Town docks, as they were about to board a steamer bound for Israel. Later on I heard that both were serving a long sentence at a Johannesburg gaol. It is remarkable to what lengths these women went to hide their identity, and I had thought their story most plausible as the parts seemed to fit together like a jigsaw puzzle.

'I have learned my lesson,' I told Alison, after the case of the bogus tourists was concluded. 'I'll not be caught out so easily again.'

Then one day a horsey-looking man swaggered into my consulting room. He was immaculately turned out in a brown-and-white sports coat, a canary-yellow waistcoat and exquisitely cut riding breeches, with boots to match. In fact he might have just walked out of Tattersalls bloodstock auctioneers! I assumed he might have been a jockey in his younger days, and now perhaps he was a trainer.

'Doc,' he said, as he sat down on the couch, 'I am suffering from a most peculiar form of indigestion. I have been having stomach pains on and off for weeks, but as they seem to be getting worse, my wife has insisted I see a doctor.'

'We live in South-West Africa,' he went on, 'some twenty miles from Windhoek, where I own a racehorse stables and stud farm. Your patient, Mr Phillips, recommended you to me. We have rented his house while he is on holiday and are staying in this area, as we wish to buy a small seaside cottage where we can spend the summer holidays and escape the arid heat of South-West Africa. But to turn to my digestive symptoms,' continued Captain Wright, 'I can't understand it. You see, when I eat something the pain goes, but when my stomach is empty again I am in pain – odd, isn't it?'

'Not a bit,' I said, 'it is typical of a duodenal ulcer: hunger pain, then the pain relieved by eating – that's just typical.'

'Well, Doc, what do you advise?'

'Although I am sure your symptoms are due to an ulcer, I should like to verify it by X-ray. If you come back tomorrow I will arrange for you to be X-rayed by a specialist in Cape Town.'

The following morning the captain returned and I was able to tell him that his X-ray appointment was for 3 p.m.

'Captain Wright,' I said, 'I have to motor into Cape Town

myself this afternoon, so if you would care to come with me, then I should be pleased to have you as a travelling companion. Why don't you come to the surgery at 2.15 p.m. and then we will set off.'

'Yes, thank you, I will see you then,' said Captain Wright. 'In fact I am just off to the station to see about a horse-van I have ordered, which I am sending up to Windhoek by goods train.' He continued, 'Oh, and before I go, Doc, I thought you might be interested in this.' Out of his coat pocket he produced a photograph. 'Have a look at this – this is me standing in front of my stables, and you can see several horses' heads peering out: real beauties, aren't they?'

I agreed that they certainly were.

'Do you know South-West Africa at all?' he enquired, as we motored into town that afternoon.

'No,' I replied, 'it has not been my good fortune to travel that far, as my family and I have only recently moved here.'

'Well,' he said, 'I have taken a liking to you, and I should be very glad if one day you would all like to come and spend a holiday with us. We have a large house set in beautiful grounds.'

'That's very kind of you,' I said, 'I am sure we would like to accept your offer one of these days.'

'This is a nice car,' enthused Captain Wright, as we drove into Cape Town.

'Yes,' I said, 'it is the new automatic Chrysler. Actually it is rather too big for me and uses too much petrol, so I am thinking of getting a smaller car for my many calls around town.'

'Are you really?' he said. 'You know, Doc, we don't see many cars like this in South-West Africa. I don't suppose you would consider selling it to me?

'Yes, of course,' I said, 'if you give me a good price and are prepared to wait until I have replaced it.' We agreed on an amount and I said, 'If you would like to come in and see me with a bank-guaranteed cheque on Monday week, I shall probably have got a smaller car by then, and I can hand this one over to you.'

'Yes, that sounds agreeable,' said Captain Wright. 'By the way, Doc, I almost forgot to tell you: I've brought one of my horses down from South-West Africa and he's running in the third race at Kenilworth this Saturday. His name is Disregard; he could probably win, but I have told my jockey to let him run second. However, on Saturday week my jockey has instructions to win – and win he will. You can put your shirt on him.'

Later I read in the *Argus* that Disregard had indeed run second, and I asked Captain Wright, 'How on earth do you arrange these things?'

'Well,' he said, 'as you know, there's a lot of dirty work in racing.' And he gave a hearty chuckle.

The captain's X-ray revealed a definite duodenal ulcer and I put him on a strict diet, including a belladonna mixture and tablets. On the Monday I expected him to bring me his cheque and take over the car. His wife, however, came instead to say that her brother-in-law, who was looking after the stables in their absence, had had a coronary thrombosis, so Captain Wright had had to fly home immediately to take over.

I have no idea where Captain Wright actually went, but I

found out later that he most certainly did not go to Windhoek. A few days later I met Mrs Wright in the town, when she asked for another prescription for her husband.

'Shall I send it directly to him in South-West Africa?' I asked.

'No,' she said, 'give it to me now, as I am writing to him today and I will enclose it with my letter.'

About ten days later Mrs Wright turned up at the surgery for another prescription and apologized that her husband's return would be further delayed.

Now, every evening on my way home from surgery I would drive past the house in which the Wrights were staying, which belonged to a Mr Phillips, and there was usually a light on in the hall and lounge. However, on this particular night the house was in total darkness and seemed completely deserted. I had a feeling that all was not as it should be, and I decided to look in on Mrs Wright in the morning and get the latest news of her husband. Imagine my surprise when I arrived at the house and was welcomed by a very excitable house-boy, who told me he himself had just returned to the house to find that 'Baas' and 'Madam' Wright had disappeared, the house was in a shocking state and that his master's bedroom, which he had locked before going on holiday, had been broken into and the contents of all the drawers taken, as well as suits stolen from his wardrobe.

'Where exactly is your Mr Phillips?' I asked him.

'He and the missus are staying at the Avalon Hotel in Montagu,' he replied.

So I phoned them up. Mr Phillips came to the phone.

'I am so sorry to trouble you, but I am phoning you about your tenants,' I said.

'Oh, such a delightful couple,' he enthused, 'and so friendly.'

'I think you may change your opinion of them when you hear what I have to say.' And I told him what had occurred in his absence.

'Good Lord,' said Mr Phillips, 'and they haven't paid a half-penny of rent.'

So unfortunately Mr and Mrs Phillips had to cut short their holiday and return to their ransacked home.

The day after my telephone call to Mr Phillips I happened to meet one of our local estate agents, who told me that he had recently shown Captain and Mrs Wright around several houses in Somerset West, in which they seemed to be interested. However, he then told me that he had just returned from a business trip to Windhoek, where to his utter astonishment he had been reliably informed that not only were there no racing stables, but that no one had ever heard of Captain and Mrs Wright.

So I quickly got busy making further enquiries. The goods office at the station denied all knowledge of a horse-van being sent to South-West Africa, and I discovered that the racehorse Disregard belonged to a well-known Cape Town businessman. How it was that the horse came in second, exactly as Captain Wright had predicted, will always remain a mystery to me.

The Criminal Investigation Department was called in and found that Captain Wright had been busily shopping in the town a few days before he and his wife did their moonlit flit, and that he had bought many pounds-worth of goods from local stores, including four new pairs of shoes. What turned out to be even more astonishing was the news that they had also stayed in a town just twenty miles away, where they had robbed the local inhabitants in exactly the same way.

Captain Wright's story was a complete fabrication; his clothes were phoney, but his image as a wealthy racehorse owner certainly paid dividends, for he was given credit wherever he went. Of course neither the specialist nor I received our medical fees. The only thing about Captain Wright that was not phoney was the fact that he genuinely had a duodenal ulcer.

I had been duped once more, and I paid the penalty for trusting such a clever pair of rogues.

IN SPRING 1950 we received the happy news that Alison was expecting our second child – although she was nearly left to raise the baby alone! I shall never forget how close I came to death one evening at a braaivleis, or South African barbecue. Some friends were talking to me and I foolishly tried to answer them and at the same time swallow a large piece of steak, which firmly lodged in my gullet, completely compressing my wind-pipe. I couldn't speak, I couldn't cough and I couldn't breathe. I was slowly suffocating and I could not make my friends under-stand the gravity of my condition. They just stared at me.

Miraculously at that moment Alison walked by and saw me put my hand to my throat. She came up and gave my back a tremendous thump – out shot the steak, and I could breathe once more. I have never before experienced such a terrible sensation: slowly suffocating and being unable to explain to bystanders the great peril I was in.

Shortly after this terrifying experience I received a telephone call from a worried maid saying, 'Please come at once, as my master can't breathe properly and he is making a horrible sound in his throat.' Within a few minutes I was round at this man's home. He was a bachelor of some sixty years and apparently after lunch he had swallowed a pill, which, instead of passing down his gullet, had entered his larynx; as he breathed in and out, the pill apparently jumped up and down, thereby interfering with his speech and breathing.

I told him to cough, but he had difficulty breathing in and consequently could not get sufficient air to blow the pill out. He was a very nervous patient, and though I banged him on the back a number of times and he tried to cough, the pill did not budge. I had visions of having to perform a tracheotomy there and then.

I decided he must be hospitalized, but as soon as the town ambulance arrived, my patient started to panic and shook his head, as if trying to say that he was not going to hospital. He then went back to his bed and lay across it facing down, with his hands on the floor, as if he was about to stand on his head. In this position he began coughing again, and I helped him with one big slap on his back – to the relief of everyone, the pill shot out and the ambulance went away empty.

On 6 January 1951 our daughter, Hazel Mary Alison, was delivered at the Edith Cavell Nursing Home, near Stellenbosch.

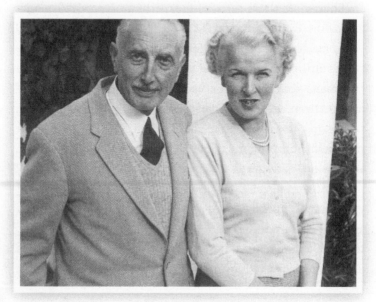

At home with Alison.

She was the only one of my children not to be born at home. In my days as a GP in Devon it was quite rare for me to attend a confinement in hospital, unless there were life-threatening circumstances. However, as time went by, home births seemed to become less fashionable.

A few years later, I discovered that Rob had inherited my fascination with snakes – an interest that could so nearly have had tragic consequences. I came home for lunch one day, after my morning surgery, and remarked to Alison that the house was extraordinarily quiet, given that Rob had a friend over to play and that they were two rather lively eleven-year-old boys. So I went to investigate, whereupon I found them in the bathroom fiddling with a shoe box which on closer scrutiny – and to my utmost horror – contained writhing baby snakes!

'Oh hello, Daddy,' Rob said cheerfully, holding one of these snakes up for me to see. 'We found these baby mole snakes under a rotten tree stump in the orchard. Jeffrey and I have each got three and we're tying them around the towel rail. Whoever's snake is the first one to drop is the loser.'

'You will both be the losers if one of these bites you!' I shouted, snatching the mustard yellow-coloured snake Rob was holding and quickly dropping it into the box. 'These are not mole snakes but baby Cape cobras – one of the deadliest snakes known to man!'

I immediately disposed of the box, sent Jeffrey home and gave Rob a hiding, warning him to stay away from all snakes until he was able to tell the difference between a harmless mole snake and a cobra!

I HAD A GREAT MANY stories about ghosts told to me when I lived in Devon, although I only ever witnessed the strange opening of that door at the haunted house that once belonged to another doctor in Dartmouth. So I was extremely curious when one of my South African patients said in passing, 'Doctor, you really should go and have a look at Garden Village – over there is a haunted house where the cups and saucers fly across the kitchen, and it is apparently the work of a poltergeist. You will find the house with ease, as there is generally a crowd around it.'

I had never witnessed this phenomenon before, so I immediately drove to the place, and sure enough when I got there the kitchen floor was littered with broken china – in fact there was not an unbroken cup or plate to be seen. The district nurse was there, and she told me that only a few minutes earlier she had been standing in the doorway of a bedroom when she saw a bottle of medicine rise in the air from a bedside table and fall at her feet. She was so scared that she beat a hasty retreat.

Poltergeist phenomena, I have since learned, are often associated with an adolescent who is mentally disturbed, and in this household there was a seventeen-year-old girl who definitely fitted the bill. A few weeks later I heard that the owner of the house had called upon a Malay priest, who had visited the house and exorcised the girl, and since then no further ghostly happenings had occurred.

'I HAVE AT LAST found my true vocation and I am now going to be a faith healer.'

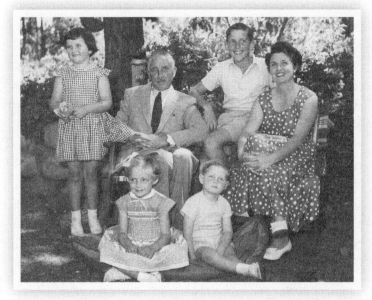

*At home in Fulmer Lodge with my children, Hazel (left), Rob and
Althea (right) and Althea's children, Tracey and Christopher.*

Leslie Bartlett was a patient of mine and a man of many talents in his varied career. He had at one time been a shop-keeper, a chicken farmer, a lawyer and a wine farmer. He was a likeable character and we had become friends, but he certainly had his eccentricities, which is why this announcement was not as surprising as it might have been.

'I've been told I have hypnotic eyes and the gift of healing,' he went on, 'and so I have decided to turn my farm into a nursing home – a haven for faith healing. I am truly sorry for you, Doc, for I don't think it will be too long before I have most of your patients recuperating at my haven.'

'Good luck to you. I hope you will soon have a large fol-lowing and a flourishing business,' I told him.

'By the way,' he went on, 'you should probably know that all my patients will be put on a very strict diet of honey, water and faith.'

'Leslie,' I suggested, 'do you think your patients will be get-ting their daily requirement of calories on your proposed diet?'

He didn't reply.

All seemed to go well with his plans until he phoned one day to tell me that he had a new patient – a diabetic – and to ask me whether it was safe to give him honey. I told him that if he did not want to aggravate his patient's condition and bring on a potential diabetic coma, then he must discontinue the honey, as honey is sugar, and sugar is the worst thing to give diabetics.

'Thanks for the advice,' he said, 'honey is obviously out.'

'But that leaves only water,' I said, 'and your patient won't get strong on that.'

'Don't forget the faith,' said my erstwhile patient.

A few days later Leslie rang again to say that he had just admitted a heart patient who had a distended abdomen and swollen legs. He thought it was dropsy – would I come out and see this patient for a consultation?

'Leslie,' I said, 'I'm afraid to say this to you, but you are a quack, and the General Medical Council forbids my association with you.'

At this Leslie was very disappointed. 'Well then,' he said, 'will you take the case over?'

'Yes,' I replied, 'if your treatment does not appear to help him, send him by ambulance to the hospital immediately and I will go and see him there.'

Apparently, though, this patient had particularly wanted a faith healer, so when there was no further improvement in his health he decided to return to his home in Hermanus, where I was told he dropped down dead the following day. I phoned Leslie and told him what a narrow escape he had had.

'What do you mean?' he asked me.

'Do you not realize that you are not allowed to issue a death certificate, should any patients die under your care? There would have to be a post-mortem, and then probably an inquiry, which at the very least would do your reputation no good at all.'

'Good heavens, I had absolutely no idea that was the case,' said Leslie.

The haven for faith healing was closed the very next day.

There have been many frauds in the business of healing, but I have always tried to keep an open mind, and I was particularly interested in the work of one well-known spiritual healer in England – a man called Harry Edwards. So much so that some years back I corresponded with him regarding my own arthritic hip, the result of an injury I sustained when helping a patient into a hospital bed many years earlier, and which continued to plague me. Many medical and religious men have dismissed Edwards, but I am not one of them. I am not entirely sure what he did, or how he did it – especially from so far away – but my hip has given me very little trouble ever since.

Perhaps the reason for my open-mindedness is in part due to my experiences as a doctor. I feel it is worth recording two cases of cancer where the sufferers refused all conventional forms of medical treatment and became completely healed, seemingly through prayer. Mrs Harris lived with her son and daughter-in-law. She was some seventy years old. One day her daughter-in-law noticed a rather unpleasant odour in the old lady's bedroom and, when Mrs Harris was questioned, she replied, 'I expect it's due to this sore on my chest.'

What she then revealed to her daughter-in-law so frightened the younger woman that she sent for me immediately.

On examining Mrs Harris I saw at once that the whole of her left breast had been eaten away and, where the breast had once been, there was now an ulcerating malignant crater measuring some three inches in diameter. This she had covered with a piece of lint onto which she had spread some Vaseline. I explained to her that the only medical treatment that might control the disease was deep X-ray treatment, though I knew her condition was quite hopeless.

She asked me if it was cancer, and I replied that unfortunately it looked as if it was.

'Well, Doctor,' she said, 'I am afraid I am not going into hospital and I refuse all medical treatment. I am going to put my trust in God and prayer, and you need not visit me again! There are frequent prayer meetings in the church to which I belong, and I shall ask all my friends to pray on my behalf.'

About a year later I was called to the same house to visit the son, who had been taken ill, and I fully expected to hear that his mother had passed away. To my amazement, I was told she was in excellent health. She came in to see me and, to my surprise, the whole ulcerated area had healed over with a thin layer of pink scar tissue, which she kept dry with boracic powder. I was naturally dumbfounded and told her so.

'Oh, Doctor, God has been very good to me,' she said, 'and all my friends rallied round me, and our united prayer has caused this miracle.'

The second case did not concern one of my patients, and I can only vouch for what I was told and actually saw. I happened to be visiting one of my bedridden patients one afternoon when I saw that she was enjoying a cup of tea with a friend.

As I entered the room the friend stood up and said, 'Well, I'll be off now, as your doctor is here.'

'No, no,' said my patient, 'please don't go, for I'm sure my doctor will be most interested in your case.' This was her friend's story.

Some eight years previously her doctor, suspecting she had a serious gynaecological condition, advised her to go and see a specialist at Groote Schuur Hospital in Cape Town. This she did and, on examination, it was found that she had inoperable cancer of the womb. The patient was offered radium and X-ray therapy, but she refused all treatment and told the doctors that the power of prayer, and her strong faith, would help her more than anything they could do.

So she returned home, and at her local church special prayer meetings were held and she herself prayed day and night. After a short time she said she began to notice a swelling in the lower right side of her abdomen. She told no one about it – it was painless, but the lump gradually increased in size and the skin over it reddened, until one day a black mass, about the size of a small apricot, burst through the skin. There was very little bleeding and she carefully dressed the wound herself every day, without informing anyone what had happened. Eventually the wound itself completely healed. Shortly afterwards she returned to Groote Schuur, was thoroughly examined and was told that her cancer of the womb had completely disappeared.

'Yes, I know,' she told the doctor, 'you will find it hard to believe, but it came out through my side.'

My patient now persuaded her friend to allow me to look at the scar, and it was grossly irregular and obviously not the work of a surgeon, but had healed very soundly. What is more, my patient's friend appeared to be in the best of health.

As I write this, I should stress that I would never advocate that an individual diagnosed with a serious illness such as cancer should refuse medical treatment; and, had this lady been my patient, I would certainly have tried to change her mind. However, I cannot ignore the possibility that her faith may well have contributed to her miraculous recovery.

During my time as a doctor I have seen many people place their faith in folk remedies. In England there was a vogue for wearing iodine lockets, which the makers claimed would ward off colds, influenza and even rheumatism. I once had a patient who used to suffer from recurring bouts of lumbago, but ever since he wore a rope around his abdomen, he declared that he had never had a recurrence. There is also a cystic condition of the tendon sheaths in the wrist, known medically as a 'ganglion'. Sufferers from this state are advised to hit it hard with a Bible to ensure it never recurs.

A patient of mine who used to suffer from sciatica told me that after he put nutmeg in his socks, this painful complaint left him. And copper bangles are supposed to cure rheumatic conditions. A Scottish lady once told me that, in her youth, bandaging a fresh herring around the neck treated tonsillitis and quinsy! Is this blind faith, or mind over matter? I do not know, but there must be some good reason for the persistence of these curious superstitions.

In South Africa applying fig juice to the skin is supposed to be a specific cure for warts. An old Afrikaner lady I once attended had a large varicose ulcer of the leg, which she was treating with the mould from the top of her home-made peach jam. She told me this was a very old Dutch remedy, used by the Afrikaner Boers for generations. When one reflects on this, she was of course using an antibiotic, for after all penicillin is a mould.

My time as a doctor in South Africa saw some of the most profound changes in our ability to heal diseases that previously were fatal, although the process had begun well before the Second World War. In 1935, when I was still practising as a GP in Devon, the first sulpha drug, Prontosil, was discovered – this was the first antibacterial drug to be made available and it was the start of a medical revolution. There followed other improvements as further sulphonamide drugs were synthesized, but for the most part these had limitations and some very unpleasant side-effects. Penicillin was discovered by Sir Alexander Fleming in 1928, but the active work was continued at Oxford by Drs Florey and Chain from about 1940 onwards. Up until this time penicillin was the only antibiotic known to be active against staphylococcus. In May 1940 scientists injected a group of mice with deadly haemolytic streptococcus – half of the group were injected with penicillin and recovered, while the other half did not receive antibiotic treatment and died.

When the Second World War broke out the quantity of penicillin available was extremely limited, so Dr Florey went to the United States and was able to secure the cooperation of the ten largest pharmaceutical companies. Soon enormous quantities of penicillin were being produced using deep-tank fermentation. By 1943 there was sufficient penicillin to meet the demand of all the Allied forces. Soon pharmaceutical companies were producing other antibiotics. Streptomycin, largely used in the treatment of tuberculosis – also known as the 'great white plague' – was isolated at Rutgers University in 1943.

The post-war years were the true era of antibiotics. In 1947 the firm of Parke-Davis produced Chloromycetin for the treatment of typhoid. In 1948 a specific against tick-bite fever – Aureomycin – was discovered by Dr Benjamin Duggar at Lederle Laboratories. Soon it became evident that some organisms were developing resistance against the antibiotics then in use, so other forms were investigated and new antibiotics were synthesized. As I write this, some 50,000 moulds have been isolated, so I hope the potential discovery of new antibiotics will lead to a limitless supply.

Although millions of lives have been saved by these wonder-drugs, some of them have alarming side-effects. There are people of an allergic disposition who are particularly sensitive to these drugs; streptomycin, for instance, has been known to cause incurable deafness and chronic vertigo. However, the relatively few who have been affected are outnumbered by the countless millions who have been saved.

As the first half of the twentieth century saw the production of life-saving antibiotics, let us hope that the second half will produce a cure for that dreaded disease – cancer.

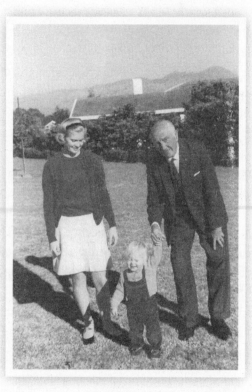

*Taking shaky steps with the help of my grandfather
in 1969 as my mother, Jennifer, looks on. She married
my father, Rob, in 1965.*

Epilogue

MY GRANDFATHER finally hung up his stethoscope in 1965, after more than half a century in medical practice. He began to pen his fascinating recollections soon afterwards and, judging by the wads of handwritten and typed notes he left behind, he clearly derived much pleasure from recalling his life's work, although I am not sure he ever envisaged them being read by anyone other than his immediate family.

He spent his retirement pursuing his interests in stamp-collecting, gardening and painting. He was a keen bridge player and was both an active member and past president of the Rotary Club of Somerset West. In 1970 he made a trip back to England, which included a sentimental visit to Dartmouth. He passed away six years later, in March 1976, aged eighty-four.

In 1983 his widow, my grandmother Alison, returned to England, where she settled in Midhurst, West Sussex. She passed away in 1988.

Althea left Kenya in 1966 and presently lives in New Zealand

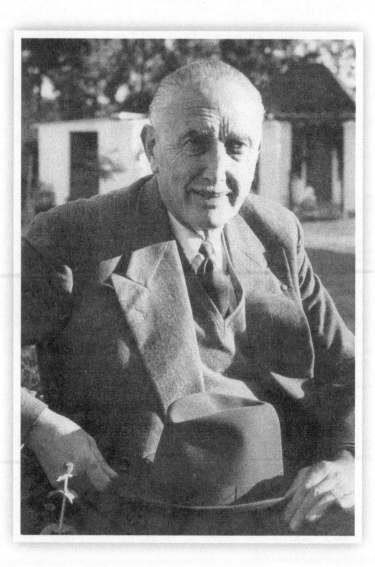

Ronald White-Cooper, 1892–1976.

with her second husband, Clarrie. She has two children, six grandchildren and seven great-grandchildren.

Rob and his wife Jenny emigrated from South Africa to the UK with their four children, including me, in 1982 and live in Virginia Water, Surrey. They have six grandchildren.

Hazel left South Africa in 1982 and lives in Newcastle, where she practises homeopathy.

ACKNOWLEDGEMENTS

ABOUT TWO YEARS AGO, I was lunching with a girlfriend, discussing how to go about getting my grandfather's stories published. A few months later, she rang to tell me that she had just been on holiday, where by chance she had met a lovely literary agent from North London who specialized in non-fiction memoirs! Jennifer Christie and I were introduced via email and it went from there.

My immense gratitude therefore goes to my dear friend Maeve McDonald for making the introduction and to Jen, who right from the word go believed in this project and has done her utmost to help make it a reality.

My sincere thanks to Ingrid Connell and her team at Macmillan for their expertise and support.

I am extremely grateful to Dr Sophie Rintoul-Hoad for her medical expertise.

Thank you to Eric Hannaford, Myra Galloway, Janet Bootherstone, Yvonne Legg, Philippa Pook, John Palmer,

Mervyn Broom and Peggy Hayes for sharing their memories of my grandfather.

To my aunt Althea and my cousin Tracey, special thanks for helping me to fill in the gaps and build the finer detail.

To my dear aunt Hazel, special thanks are due for her enthusiasm and encouragement.

My heartfelt appreciation to my wonderful parents Rob and Jen, my sisters Lib and Cath, and my brother Steve for their unfaltering love and support in all I do.

To Georgia and Sam, huge hugs for your patience and for allowing Mummy time and space to finish this book!